Sleep in Older Adults

Editors

CATHY A. ALESSI
JENNIFER L. MARTIN

SLEEP MEDICINE CLINICS

www.sleep.theclinics.com

Consulting Editor
TEOFILO LEE-CHIONG Jr

March 2018 • Volume 13 • Number 1

ELSEVIER

1600 John F. Kennedy Boulevard • Suite 1800 • Philadelphia, Pennsylvania, 19103-2899

http://www.theclinics.com

SLEEP MEDICINE CLINICS Volume 13, Number 1
March 2018, ISSN 1556-407X, ISBN-13: 978-0-323-58174-5

Editor: Colleen Dietzler
Developmental Editor: Donald Mumford

Sleep Medicine Clinics (ISSN 1556-407X) is published quarterly by Elsevier Inc., 360 Park Avenue South, New York, NY 10010-1710. Months of issue are March, June, September and December. Business and Editorial Offices: 1600 John F. Kennedy Blvd., Ste. 1800, Philadelphia, PA 19103-2899. Customer Service Office: 3251 Riverport Lane, Maryland Heights, MO 63043. Periodicals postage paid at New York, NY and additional mailing offices. Subscription prices are $203.00 per year (US individuals), $100.00 (US students), $486.00 (US institutions), $245.00 (Canadian and international individuals), $135.00 (Canadian and international students), $540.00 (Canadian institutions) and $540.00 (International institutions). Foreign air speed delivery is included in all *Clinics* subscription prices. All prices are subject to change without notice. **POSTMASTER:** Send change of address to *Sleep Medicine Clinics*, Elsevier Health Sciences Division, Subscription Customer Service, 3251 Riverport Lane, Maryland Heights, MO 63043. Customer Service: **Tel: 1-800-654-2452 (U.S. and Canada); 314-447-8871 (outside U.S. and Canada). Fax: 314-447-8029. E-mail: journalscustomerservice-usa@elsevier.com (for print support); journalsonlinesupport-usa@elsevier.com (for online support).**

Reprints. For copies of 100 or more of articles in this publication, please contact the Commercial Reprints Department, Elsevier Inc., 360 Park Avenue South, New York, NY 10010-1710. Tel.: 212-633-3874; Fax: 212-633-3820; E-mail: reprints@elsevier.com.

Sleep Medicine Clinics is covered in *MEDLINE/PubMed (Index Medicus)*.

PROGRAM OBJECTIVE

The goal of *Sleep Medicine Clinics of North America* is to keep practicing physicians up to date with current clinical practice by providing timely articles reviewing the state of the art in patient care.

TARGET AUDIENCE

All practicing physicians and other healthcare professionals.

LEARNING OBJECTIVES

Upon completion of this activity, participants will be able to:
1. Review typical and atypical sleep patterns in the aging adult.
2. Discuss the effects of chronic medical conditions on sleep.
3. Recognize considerations for sleep in hospitalized and long term care patients.

ACCREDITATION

The Elsevier Office of Continuing Medical Education (EOCME) is accredited by the Accreditation Council for Continuing Medical Education (ACCME) to provide continuing medical education for physicians.

The EOCME designates this enduring material for a maximum of 15 *AMA PRA Category 1 Credit*(s)™. Physicians should claim only the credit commensurate with the extent of their participation in the activity.

All other healthcare professionals requesting continuing education credit for this enduring material will be issued a certificate of participation.

DISCLOSURE OF CONFLICTS OF INTEREST

The EOCME assesses conflict of interest with its instructors, faculty, planners, and other individuals who are in a position to control the content of CME activities. All relevant conflicts of interest that are identified are thoroughly vetted by EOCME for fair balance, scientific objectivity, and patient care recommendations. EOCME is committed to providing its learners with CME activities that promote improvements or quality in healthcare and not a specific proprietary business or a commercial interest.

The planning committee, staff, authors and editors listed below have identified no financial relationships or relationships to products or devices they or their spouse/life partner have with commercial interest related to the content of this CME activity:
Vineet M. Arora, MD, MAPP; M. Safwan Badr, MD; Glenna S. Brewster, PhD, RN, FNP-BC; Susmita Chowdhuri, MD, MS; Joseph Daniel; Colleen Dietzler; Christopher W. Drapeau, PhD; Jeanne F. Duffy, MBA, PhD; Anjali Fortna; Philip R. Gehrman, PhD, CBSM; Nalaka S. Gooneratne, MD, MSc; Alex Iranzo, MD; Jee Hyun Kim, MD, PhD; Teofilo Lee-Chiong Jr, MD; Junxin Li, PhD; Leah Logan; Raman K. Malhotra, MD; Michael R. Nadorff, PhD; Saban-Hakki Onen, MD, PhD; Fannie Onen, MD, PhD; Pragnesh Patel, MD; Wilfred R. Pigeon, PhD; Scott Ravyts, MS; Kathy C. Richards, PhD, RN, FAAN; Barbara Riegel, PhD, RN; Nancy H. Stewart, DO; Camille P. Vaughan, MD, MS; Michael V. Vitiello, PhD; Lichuan Ye, PhD, RN.

The planning committee, staff, authors and editors listed below have identified financial relationships or relationships to products or devices they or their spouse/life partner have with commercial interest related to the content of this CME activity:
Donald L. Bliwise, PhD has research support from New England Research Institutes, and receives royalties/patents from Ferring Pharmaceuticals; Merck & Co., Inc.; and Vantia Therapeutics Ltd.
Natalie Dautovich, PhD is a consultant/advisor for the National Sleep Foundation and Merck & Co., Inc.
Joseph M. Dzierzewski, PhD has research support from the National Institute on Aging.

UNAPPROVED/OFF-LABEL USE DISCLOSURE

The EOCME requires CME faculty to disclose to the participants:
1. When products or procedures being discussed are off-label, unlabelled, experimental, and/or investigational (not US Food and Drug Administration [FDA] approved); and
2. Any limitations on the information presented, such as data that are preliminary or that represent ongoing research, interim analyses, and/or unsupported opinions. Faculty may discuss information about pharmaceutical agents that is outside of FDA-approved labelling. This information is intended solely for CME and is not intended to promote off-label use of these medications. If you have any questions, contact the medical affairs department of the manufacturer for the most recent prescribing information.

TO ENROLL

To enroll in the Sleep Medicine Clinics Continuing Medical Education program, call customer service at 1-800-654-2452 or sign up online at http://www.theclinics.com/home/cme. The CME program is available to subscribers for an additional annual fee of USD $140.

METHOD OF PARTICIPATION

In order to claim credit, participants must complete the following:

1. Complete enrolment as indicated above.
2. Read the activity.
3. Complete the CME Test and Evaluation. Participants must achieve a score of 70% on the test. All CME Tests and Evaluations must be completed online.

CME INQUIRIES/SPECIAL NEEDS

For all CME inquiries or special needs, please contact elsevierCME@elsevier.com.

SLEEP MEDICINE CLINICS

THE CLINICS ARE AVAILABLE ONLINE!
Access your subscription at:
www.theclinics.com

Contributors

CONSULTING EDITOR

TEOFILO LEE-CHIONG Jr, MD
Professor of Medicine, National Jewish Health,
University of Colorado Denver, Denver,
Colorado; Chief Medical Liaison, Philips
Respironics, Pennsylvania, USA

EDITORS

CATHY A. ALESSI, MD
Director, Geriatric Research, Education and
Clinical Center, VA Greater Los Angeles
Healthcare System, Professor, David Geffen
School of Medicine at UCLA, Los Angeles,
California, USA

JENNIFER L. MARTIN, PhD
Associate Director, Clinical and Health
Services Research, Geriatric Research,
Education and Clinical Center, VA Greater
Los Angeles Healthcare System, Associate
Professor, David Geffen School of Medicine at
UCLA, Los Angeles, California, USA

AUTHORS

VINEET M. ARORA, MD, MAPP
Associate Professor, Department of
Medicine, The University of Chicago, Chicago,
Illinois, USA

M. SAFWAN BADR, MD
Sleep Medicine Section, John D. Dingell VA
Medical Center, Department of Medicine,
Wayne State University, Detroit, Michigan,
USA

DONALD L. BLIWISE, PhD
Professor, Program in Sleep, Aging
and Chronobiology, Department of
Neurology, Emory University, Atlanta, Georgia,
USA

GLENNA S. BREWSTER, PhD, RN, FNP-BC
Research Assistant Professor,
Nell Hodgson Woodruff School of
Nursing, Emory University, Atlanta, Georgia,
USA; Center for Sleep and Circadian
Neurobiology, Perelman School of Medicine
University of Pennsylvania, Philadelphia,
Pennsylvania, USA

SUSMITA CHOWDHURI, MD, MS
Sleep Medicine Section, John D. Dingell VA
Medical Center, Department of Medicine,
Wayne State University, Detroit, Michigan,
USA

NATALIE DAUTOVICH, PhD
Assistant Professor, Department of
Psychology, Virginia Commonwealth
University, Richmond, Virginia, USA

CHRISTOPHER W. DRAPEAU, PhD
Postdoctoral Fellow, Department of
Psychology, Mississippi State University,
Mississippi State, Mississippi, USA; Assistant
Professor, Department of Education,
Valparaiso University, Valparaiso, Indiana, USA

JEANNE F. DUFFY, MBA, PhD
Associate Professor of Medicine, Division of
Sleep and Circadian Disorders, Departments
of Medicine and Neurology, Brigham and
Women's Hospital, Division of Sleep Medicine,
Harvard Medical School, Boston,
Massachusetts, USA

JOSEPH M. DZIERZEWSKI, PhD
Assistant Professor, Department
of Psychology, Virginia Commonwealth
University, Richmond, Virginia, USA

PHILIP R. GEHRMAN, PhD, CBSM
Center for Sleep and Circadian
Neurobiology, Department of Psychiatry,
Perelman School of Medicine University
of Pennsylvania, Philadelphia, Pennsylvania,
USA

NALAKA S. GOONERATNE, MD, MSc
Geriatrics Division, Perelman School
of Medicine, University of Pennsylvania,
Associate Professor, Center for Sleep
and Circadian Neurobiology, Philadelphia,
Pennsylvania, USA

ALEX IRANZO, MD
Neurology Service, Multidisciplinary Sleep
Unit, Hospital Clinic de Barcelona, Barcelona,
Spain

JEE HYUN KIM, MD, PhD
Associate Professor, Department
of Neurology, Dankook University College
of Medicine, Dankook University Hospital,
Cheonan, Chungnam, Republic of Korea;
Visiting Scientist, Division of Sleep and
Circadian Disorders, Departments of
Medicine and Neurology, Brigham and
Women's Hospital, Division of Sleep Medicine,
Harvard Medical School, Boston,
Massachusetts, USA

JUNXIN LI, PhD
Postdoctoral Research Fellow,
Center for Sleep and Circadian
Neurobiology, School of Nursing, Perelman
School of Medicine University
of Pennsylvania, Philadelphia, Pennsylvania,
USA

RAMAN K. MALHOTRA, MD
Associate Professor, Department
of Neurology, Saint Louis University
School of Medicine, St Louis, Missouri,
USA

MICHAEL R. NADORFF, PhD
Assistant Professor, Department of
Psychology, Mississippi State University,
Mississippi State, Mississippi, USA; Adjunct
Assistant Professor, Menninger Department of
Psychiatry and Behavioral Sciences, Baylor
College of Medicine, Houston, Texas, USA

FANNIE ONEN, MD, PhD
Department of Geriatrics, Bichat University
Hospital, APHP, INSERM 1178 and CESP,
University of Paris-Sud, Paris, France

SABAN-HAKKI ONEN, MD, PhD
Geriatric Sleep Medicine Center, Eduard
Herriot University Hospital, HCL, INSERM
1028, University of Lyon, Lyon, France

PRAGNESH PATEL, MD
Department of Medicine, Wayne State
University, Detroit, Michigan, USA

WILFRED R. PIGEON, PhD
Associate Professor, Department of
Psychiatry, University of Rochester, Rochester,
New York, USA; Director, VISN 2 Center of
Excellence for Suicide Prevention,
Canandaigua VA Medical Center,
Canandaigua, New York, USA

SCOTT RAVYTS, MS
Graduate Student, Department of Psychology,
Virginia Commonwealth University, Richmond,
Virginia, USA

KATHY C. RICHARDS, PhD, RN, FAAN
Research Professor, The University of Texas at
Austin, School of Nursing, Austin, Texas, USA

BARBARA RIEGEL, PhD, RN
University of Pennsylvania School of Nursing,
Philadelphia, Pennsylvania, USA

NANCY H. STEWART, DO
Fellow, Creighton University Medical Center,
Omaha, Nebraska, USA

CAMILLE P. VAUGHAN, MD, MS
Investigator, Birmingham/Atlanta Geriatric
Research, Education, and Clinical Center,
Atlanta VA Health Care System, Decatur,
Georgia, USA; Assistant Professor, Division of
General Medicine and Geriatrics, Department
of Medicine, Emory University, Atlanta,
Georgia, USA

MICHAEL V. VITIELLO, PhD
Professor, Department of Psychiatry and
Behavioral Sciences, University of Washington,
Seattle, Washington, USA

LICHUAN YE, PhD, RN
Associate Professor, Bouvé College of Health
Sciences, Northeastern University, Boston,
Massachusetts, USA

Contents

Parasomnias and Sleep-Related Movement Disorders in Older Adults

Alex Iranzo

Neurodegenerative Disorders and Sleep

Raman K. Malhotra

Chronic Medical Conditions and Sleep in the Older Adult

Saban-Hakki Onen and Fannie Onen

Psychiatric Illness and Sleep in Older Adults: Comorbidity and Opportunities for Intervention

Michael R. Nadorff, Christopher W. Drapeau, and Wilfred R. Pigeon

Preface

Sleep in Older Adults: Challenges and Opportunities

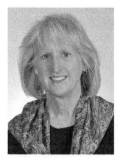 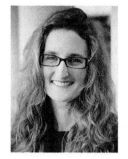

Cathy A. Alessi, MD   Jennifer L. Martin, PhD
Editors

Sleep problems are common among older adults, can significantly impact health and quality of life, and can present unique challenges for diagnosis and management. This series of articles provides a state-of-the-art, evidence-based review of key topics in the assessment and management of sleep problems in older adults. Written by leading experts in various fields, from around the United States and internationally, these articles address changes in sleep that occur with healthy aging and illness, in addition to important and unique issues clinicians must consider when caring for the older adult with disturbed sleep.

In the first article, Li, Vitiello, and Gooneratne provide a careful review of clinically relevant age-related changes in sleep and circadian rhythms, particularly advanced sleep timing, decreased slow-wave sleep, shortened nighttime sleep duration, increased nighttime awakenings and time spent awake at night, and increased frequency of daytime napping. Interestingly, most of these and other age-related changes in sleep occur by middle age, with sleep remaining relatively stable after 60 years of age in healthy older adults. Aging is also associated with less robust circadian rhythms and sleep homeostasis, which contribute to sleep changes with aging. In addition, age-related changes in neuroendocrine functions contribute to or correlate with alterations of sleep quality and architecture in normal aging. Finally, the authors describe the multifactorial nature of sleep disturbance in older adults, including common medical comorbidities and psychiatric illnesses, primary sleep disorders, and changes in social engagement, lifestyle, and environment that can play a role in sleep.

Brewster, Riegel, and Gehrman provide an overview of insomnia disorder in older adults, highlighting different types of insomnia complaints (ie, difficulty falling asleep at the start of the sleep period, waking up during the night and having difficulty falling back asleep, and waking up early and being unable to get back to sleep), and how the types of insomnia complaints in older people differ from their younger counterparts. Given the medical and psychiatric complexity of many older adults, they also highlight the importance of a thorough medical history in evaluating older people with difficulties sleeping. Finally, they discuss treatment of insomnia in older patients, highlighting the benefits achieved with cognitive behavioral therapy for insomnia, a multicomponent treatment including stimulus control, sleep restriction, sleep hygiene, and cognitive therapy, as the recommended first-line therapy for treatment of insomnia in older adults. They also discuss the potential risks in older adults (eg, falls) associated with many pharmacologic agents used to manage insomnia.

Sleep Med Clin 13 (2018) xv–xviii
https://doi.org/10.1016/j.jsmc.2017.12.002
1556-407X/18/© 2017 Published by Elsevier Inc.

sleep.theclinics.com

Sleep apnea or sleep-disordered breathing (SDB) is another common sleep disorder in older people. In their article, Chowdhuri, Patel, and Badr review the spectrum of age-related considerations in SDB, from pathophysiology to treatment. Older patients have higher rates of SDB, and in particular, higher rates of central apneas. In addition, the risks for cardiovascular, metabolic, and neurocognitive sequelae when SDB is left untreated are particularly important in the older population. While the treatment of choice for SDB is positive airway pressure therapy, and available studies show that older patients do benefit from treatment, the authors highlight that research in this area is needed. They also note that studies of other therapies for SDB have not been conducted with older patients. Future research on the challenges and benefits of treating SDB in older patients is still needed.

Kim and Duffy discuss how the circadian timing system changes with advancing age, including the natural shift of internal circadian rhythms to an earlier time, and a decreased ability of older adults to shift the timing of their circadian clock. They bring this discussion into clinical application, highlighting the reasons older adults suffer from higher rates of circadian rhythm sleep disorders, such as advanced sleep-wake phase disorder and irregular sleep-wake rhythm disorder, leading to sleep-related complaints and reduced quality of life. They also discuss why older adults are more prone to jet lag disorder and shift work disorder because of alterations in the circadian timing system.

In the next article, Iranzo reviews rapid eye movement (REM) sleep behavior disorder and other parasomnias in the older adult, which are important and interesting problems in this population. First, disorders of arousal from non-REM (NREM) sleep, such as sleepwalking and sleep terrors, are discussed, since these conditions may persist in the older adult. In addition, medications (such as zolpidem and other agents) may induce sleepwalking and sleep-related eating, including among older people. The article provides a particularly comprehensive and state-of-the-art review of REM sleep behavior disorder, which is particularly important in older adults. Individuals with idiopathic REM sleep behavior disorder represent a prodromal stage of Parkinson disease and related synucleinopathies. In addition, a careful description is provided for anti-IgLON5 disease, which is an interesting and novel condition characterized by abnormal sleep architecture, abnormal behaviors in NREM sleep, and REM sleep behavior disorder. This condition is characterized by antibodies against the protein IgLON5, the presence of HLA-DQB1*05:01, and tau deposits involving the brainstem and the hypothalamus. Finally, restless legs syndrome and periodic limb movements in sleep are reviewed, particularly in terms of unique aspects of these conditions in older adults.

The next article, by Malhotra, provides a comprehensive and enlightening review of neurodegenerative disorders and sleep. Sleep problems are commonly found in older adults with neurodegenerative disorders, such as Parkinson's disease and Alzheimer's disease, and the clinician managing sleep problems in older adults needs a thorough understanding of these conditions. The sleep disorders identified may be due to the primary symptoms of the neurodegenerative disease itself or may result from damage to sleep-controlling centers in the brain. Common sleep disorders found in this population include insomnia, hypersomnia, sleep apnea, restless legs syndrome, circadian rhythm disorders, and REM sleep behavior disorder. As mentioned above, REM sleep behavior disorder can present years before any other neurologic symptoms or signs are present, serving as a precursor to Parkinson's disease or other synucleinopathies. Of keen interest is the growing evidence that poor sleep can lead to acceleration in the progression of neurodegenerative disorders and may play a role in the pathogenesis of these potentially devastating conditions.

Sleep problems in older adults commonly occur in the setting of complex comorbidity, and, in the next article, Onen and Onen provide an informative review of the evidence for a relationship between medical conditions and sleep in the older adult. Since older adults with sleep disturbances and chronic medical conditions may have tremendous clinical heterogeneity and complexity, the management of sleep disturbances in older age can be both challenging and fascinating. Pain and sleep disturbance is an important example, since the pain itself, the underlying disease process(es) causing pain, and medication to treat pain, can all disturb sleep. The relationship is also bidirectional, since sleep disturbances may adversely affect the natural course of chronic painful disease in older adults. With cancer, in particular, sleep disturbance may negatively affect the patient's experience by increasing fatigue and discomfort, and reducing emotional well-being. Increased risk of falls in older adults is another area of importance to the clinician interested in sleep. Falls are common in older adults with insomnia and sleep apnea, and sedative hypnotics increase the risk of falls. The relationship between sleep apnea and heart disease, as it relates to older adults, is also addressed. In particular, heart failure may contribute to sleep apnea through a variety of mechanisms, and sleep apnea may impair cardiac function chronically by increasing sympathetic activity and oxidative stress leading to increased blood pressure, nocturnal arrhythmias, and stroke.

Comorbid psychiatric illness has a significant impact on sleep in older adults. Nadorff, Drapeau, and Pigeon explore the association between sleep disorders and psychopathology among older adults and note similarities in the relationship between poor sleep and anxiety, depression, dementia, and suicidal behavior. They discuss literature related to high rates of comorbid psychiatric disorders in patients with sleep disorders and vice versa. They also discuss important findings related to sleep disruption as a suicide risk factor among older adults, even beyond the effects of psychopathology. The authors note a need for research examining the potential benefits of treating sleep disorders on psychiatric symptoms specifically in older people.

In an excellent review of the literature on sleep and cognition in older adults, Dzierzewski, Dautovich, and Ravyts discuss both normative changes in cognition and cognitive decline associated with pathology. They report that negative changes in sleep are associated with worse cognitive functioning, and that is true across subgroups of older patients, including those with and without sleep disorders. They focus on cognitive correlates of both insomnia and SDB, noting that evidence is mixed regarding the benefits of treatment. Some studies have shown cognitive benefits associated with treatment of insomnia and SDB, while other studies have not. They conclude by noting that understanding the mechanisms through which sleep can improve cognitive functioning in older people may facilitate development of promising new interventions.

No review of sleep problems in older adults would be complete without addressing the topic of sleep and nocturia, which is provided in a thoughtful and practical format in the article by Vaughan and Bliwise. Older people frequently experience nocturia and sleep disturbance concurrently, and problems with sleep resulting

from nocturia are a major factor associated with the degree of bother (or discomfort) that older people attribute to nocturia. Nocturia among older adults is often the result of multiple chronic conditions or predisposing factors, so a multi-component treatment strategy is usually warranted. Initial treatment includes lifestyle modification and behavioral treatment with consideration of pelvic floor muscle exercise–based therapy. Behavioral treatment for nocturia appears to provide a reduction in nocturia that is similar to the most frequently used drug therapies for nocturia. Medication-based treatments for nocturia available include alpha-blockers and bladder relaxants; the role of other agents, such as antidiuretic therapy, remains uncertain. If initial treatment strategies for nocturia do not provide significant improvement, a more formal sleep evaluation should be considered in the older adult with nocturia, since certain sleep disorders, such as sleep apnea and restless legs syndrome, may predispose and/or contribute to nocturia.

Many older adults will spend some portion of their later years in an institutional long-term care (LTC) facility, and while many of the same factors that disrupt sleep in community settings also disrupt sleep in LTC, there are additional issues to consider. Ye and Richards note that poor sleep increases risk for LTC placement, and sleep disturbance is extremely common among LTC residents. They discuss challenges in the evaluation and diagnosis of sleep disorders, such as insomnia, SDB, and restless legs syndrome, and suggest that management of sleep disturbance in LTC residents is an important aspect of offering high-quality care for this already compromised population. In addition, they provide recommendations for how to improve sleep quality among LTC residents using nonpharmacologic strategies.

Finally, Stewart and Arora provide an evidence-based review of sleep in the hospitalized older adult. Older adults make up the majority of hospitalized patients, and hospitalization is typically a period of acute sleep deprivation for older adults due to environmental, medical, and patient factors. Although hospitalized patients are likely in need of adequate rest to aid in their recovery during acute illness, these patients face unique risks due to the acute sleep loss of hospitalization. Evidence suggests that sleep loss in the hospital is associated with worse health outcomes, including cardiometabolic derangements and increased risk of delirium. Because older patients are at risk of polypharmacy and medication side effects, non-pharmacologic interventions are recommended as the first-line choice to improve sleep in hospitalized older adults.

We greatly appreciate the hard work and dedication of these authors in providing practical, evidence-based reviews of key topics related to sleep in older adults. As described in these pages, sleep disturbance can significantly impact the health and well-being of older adults, and complex medical and psychiatric comorbidity often plays a key role in understanding and managing sleep problems in this population. To quote Ralph Waldo Emerson, "Health is the first muse, and sleep is the condition to produce it." We hope this work will provide useful and timely guidance for clinicians and will spark interest in researchers, educators, and others to address the important and unique issues that must be considered when caring for the older adult with disturbed sleep.

Cathy A. Alessi, MD
Geriatric Research, Education and Clinical Center
VA Greater Los Angeles Healthcare System
David Geffen School of Medicine
at the University of California, Los Angeles
Los Angeles, CA 91343, USA

Jennifer L. Martin, PhD
Geriatric Research, Education and Clinical Center
VA Greater Los Angeles Healthcare System
David Geffen School of Medicine
at the University of California, Los Angeles
Los Angeles, CA 91343, USA

E-mail addresses:
cathy.alessi@va.gov (C.A. Alessi)
jennifer.martin@va.gov (J.L. Martin)

Sleep in Normal Aging

Junxin Li, PhD[a,b,]*, Michael V. Vitiello, PhD[c],
Nalaka S. Gooneratne, MD, MSc[d]

KEYWORDS

- Sleep architecture • Circadian rhythm • Sleep homeostasis • Hormone • Normal aging

KEY POINTS

- Age-related changes in sleep include advanced sleep timing, shortened nocturnal sleep duration, increased frequency of daytime naps, increased nocturnal awakenings and time spent awake, and decreased slow wave sleep.
- Most age-related changes in sleep are stable after 60 years of age among older adults with excellent health.
- Aging is associated with less robust circadian rhythms and sleep homeostasis, which contribute to sleep changes in aging.
- Age-related changes in neuroendocrine functions contribute to or correlate with alterations of sleep quality and architecture in normal aging.
- Multiple factors, including medical comorbidities and psychiatric illness, primary sleep disorders, and changes in social engagement, lifestyle, and environment contribute to sleep disturbances in older adults.

INTRODUCTION

Sleep has received increasing attention within the context of geriatric research based on a growing body of evidence that links poor sleep with many adverse health outcomes, especially decline in cognition, in older adults. Along with many other physiologic alterations in normal aging, sleep patterns change with aging, independent of many factors, including medical comorbidity and medications.[1] Total sleep time (TST), sleep efficiency, and deep sleep (slow wave sleep) decrease with aging, and the number of nocturnal awakenings and time spent awake during the night increase with aging.[2] These age-related changes in sleep are associated not only with changes in the circadian and homeostatic processes, but also with some normal physiologic and psychosocial changes in aging. This article describes age-related changes in sleep, circadian rhythms, and sleep-related hormones. We focus on changes associated with normal aging rather than changes that accompany common pathologic processes in older adults, which are discussed in detail elsewhere.

AGE-RELATED CHANGES IN SLEEP

There is no doubt that sleep changes as a function of age.[3] Aging is associated with decreased ability to maintain sleep (increased number of awakenings and prolonged nocturnal awakenings), reduced nocturnal sleep duration, and decreased deep sleep (slow wave sleep).[4] Herein we discuss in detail age-related changes in sleep duration, sleep initiation, sleep efficiency, sleep maintenance, sleep stages, daytime sleep behaviors, and self-reported sleep quality. An important aspect of this discussion is to differentiate

Disclosure Statement: N/A.
[a] School of Nursing, University of Pennsylvania, Philadelphia, PA 19104, USA; [b] Center for Sleep and Circadian Neurobiology, Perelman School of Medicine, University of Pennsylvania, 3624 Market Street, Philadelphia, PA 19104, USA; [c] Department of Psychiatry and Behavioral Sciences, University of Washington, Box 356560, Seattle, WA 98195-6560, USA; [d] Geriatrics Division, Perelman School of Medicine, University of Pennsylvania, Center for Sleep and Circadian Neurobiology, 3615 Chestnut Street, Philadelphia, PA 19104, USA
* Corresponding author.
E-mail address: junxin.li@uphs.upenn.edu

sleep.theclinics.com

changes in sleep that occur from childhood to age 60 (or 65), versus those that occur after this point. Ohayon and colleagues[2] comprehensively reviewed the normative sleep changes from childhood to old age using metaanalysis results from 65 studies (polysomnography or actigraphy) representing 3577 healthy subjects aged between 5 and 102 years of age, and this work informs many of the insights discussed in this review. Older subjects (defined as age >60 years) in this analysis were more representative of older adults with excellent health and who were optimally aging, rather than the general older adult population.[4]

Sleep Duration

The current literature supports that, in general, the TST decreases with age (from pediatric to older adulthood). However, further age-associated decreases in TST have not been observed consistently after entering older age brackets. Campbell and colleagues[5] in 2007 conducted a laboratory study with 50 healthy adults aged between 19 and 81 years to evaluate the spontaneous sleep across the 24-hour day among young, middle-aged, and older adults. Compared with young adults (10.5 hours), middle-aged (9.1 hours) and older adults (8.1 hours) had significantly shorter average nighttime sleep duration. Data from 160 healthy adults (without sleep complaints) aged between 20 and 90 years from the SIESTA database showed that TST decreased about 8 minutes per decade in males and 10 minutes per decade in females.[6] Similarly, 3 metaanalysis reviews reported that age was linearly associated with decreased TST, with an approximately 10- to 12-minute reduction per decade of age in the adult population.[2,7,8] This association was stronger when comparing young adults with middle-aged or older adults, but vanished within older subjects who were 60 years of age and older. These findings indicate that TST plateaued after 60 years of age. Also, the association was stronger in women than men.[2]

Sleep Initiation

People commonly assume that the ability to initiate sleep decreases significantly with age. However, current evidence does not support this assumption, but suggests that both sleep latency and the ability to fall back to sleep after nocturnal awakenings demonstrate minimal increases after the age of 60 years. Results from 2 metaanalyses, for example, suggest that sleep latency does increase with age. However, the magnitude of change is very modest.[2,8] In these studies, sleep latency holds constant from childhood to

adolescence. The significant age-related increase in sleep latency was only found between very young adults and older adults. A mathematical modeling, which was conducted using data from 7 laboratory sleep studies (258 subjects aged 17–91 years), suggested that sleep latency increased between the late teens and 20s, remains constant from age 30 until approximate age 50 years, and then increased steadily after age 50 years.[9] However, the amount or magnitude of changes were not reported. In addition, even though more frequent arousals were found in healthy older adults than young people, older adults maintained their ability to reinitiate sleep and fell back to sleep as rapidly as younger adults.[3,10]

Sleep Efficiency

Sleep efficiency remains largely unchanged from childhood to adolescence and significantly decreases with age in adulthood. Different from all other sleep parameters that hold steady after 60 years of age, sleep efficiency continues to decline very slowly with advancing age.[2]

Sleep Maintenance

Aging from birth to older adulthood is associated with a decreased ability to maintain sleep, which presents as the increased number of arousals (arousal index) and longer duration of wake after sleep onset (WASO), but also tends to plateau after age 60.[2,8] In the metaanalysis performed by Ohayon and colleagues,[2] age-related change in WASO achieved the largest effect size among all sleep parameters, which yielded a steady 10 minutes increase of WASO per decade of age from 30 to 60 years. WASO remained mostly unchanged after age 60 years.

Sleep Stages

In general, deep sleep (slow wave sleep) decreases with age in the adult population. During nocturnal sleep, the proportion of non–rapid eye movement sleep stage 1 and stage 2 increases with age, and the proportion of slow-wave sleep and rapid eye movement sleep (REM) sleep decreases with age[2,11] (Fig. 1). These changes were not significant among healthy older adults aged more than 60 years.[2] Also, the association between age and decreased REM latency was minimal.[2] Floyd and colleagues's[7] metaanalysis reported a linear decrease in the proportion of REM with a small rate of 0.6% per decade from age 19 until 75 years of age, then small increases were found in the proportion of REM between 75 and 85 years of age.

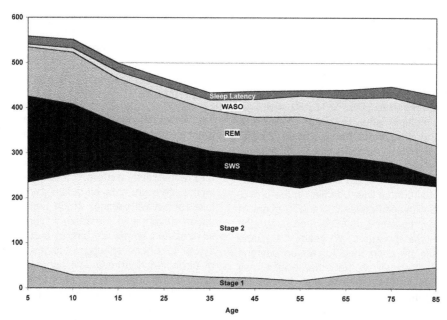

Fig. 1. Age-related changes in sleep architecture. REM, rapid eye movement; SWS, slow wave sleep; WASO, wake after sleep onset. (*From* Ohayon MM, Carskadon MA, Guilleminault C, et al. Meta-analysis of quantitative sleep parameters from childhood to old age in healthy individuals: developing normative sleep values across the human lifespan. Sleep 2004;27(7):1255–73.)

There may be gender differences in age-related changes in sleep stages. The metaanalysis conducted by Ohayon and colleagues suggested that the age effect on the percentage of stage 1 sleep was stronger in women, and women had less percentage of stage 2 sleep and a greater percentage of slow wave sleep than age-matched men. The SIESTA study found that women had no change in slow wave sleep with age, in contrast with men, who had a 1.7% decrease in slow wave sleep per decade of age. In addition, women had a smaller rate of increase in stage 1 sleep, a greater rate of increase in stage 2 sleep, and a greater rate of decline in REM, in comparison with men.[6] These results indicate that men may be more prone to age-related decline in slow wave sleep than women.

Daytime Napping and Daytime Sleepiness

Daytime napping is a daily routine for many people across the lifespan. Results from epidemiology studies suggest that daytime napping is more prevalent in older adults than that seen in younger adults.[12–15] Several studies have found that older adults nap more frequently than younger and middle-aged adults,[14,16,17] this is also true when comparing healthy older adults with younger individuals.[18] Within the older population, 1 study found that nap frequency increased with age.[19] A recent study using 7664 people, aged 20 to 99 years, from a national representative sample in Japan, found that a higher proportion of older adults (27.4%) take frequent naps (≥4 d/wk) than young (11.9%) and middle-aged (14.4%) adults.[14] However, no clear evidence supports that nap duration is different between older adults and other adult populations.[5,19] A laboratory study by Campbell and colleagues[5] in 2007 showed that nap durations were not different among the young, middle-aged, and older adults, but that the number of daytime naps increased with age. Yoon and colleagues[18] reported that older adults tended to nap at a different time than younger adults, where older adults were more likely to nap in the early evening, whereas younger adults were more likely to nap in the afternoon.[20]

People choose to take a nap for many reasons, such as to compensate for nighttime sleep loss, to restore energy and reduce daytime sleepiness, or just to relax.[20] Cultural background also has a considerable influence on nap habits. For example, midday naps are a common practice of people from China, and Mediterranean and several Latin American countries.[21] Older adults may nap more frequently owing to both biological changes, but also to lifestyle changes that accompany aging. For example, older adults may spend less time on work and physical and social activities, and thus have more opportunities to nap than young and middle-aged adults during the day. Also, Foley and colleagues[22] found that frequent napping was associated with excessive daytime sleepiness (EDS), depression, pain and nocturia in a U. nationally representative poll of older adults.

Epidemiologic studies indicated that up to 20% of older adults reported EDS.[23–26] EDS usually coexists with multiple adverse health conditions, including cognitive impairment, cardiovascular events, and increased mortality risk.[27,28] Certainly, EDS is not a part of normal aging, but may be a signal or symptom of certain diseases. An epidemiologic study found a linear decline in the prevalence of EDS with age between 30 and 75 years. In addition, the prevalence of EDS decreased at a greater rate after the age of 75 years.[29] Daytime napping could be a practice to reduce daytime sleepiness[15]; however, some older adults may experience daytime sleepiness but do not fall asleep during the day.[26]

Self-Reported Sleep Quality

People may expect that older adults complain more about their sleep than younger aged adults because most objectively measured sleep parameters decrease with age. However, this may not be the case; there can be significant differences between objective and self-reported perceptions of sleep, and comorbidities can play a major role. For example, although some epidemiologic studies found that up to 50% of older adults have self-reported poor sleep,[30,31] a large proportion of these complaints are attributable to older adults' poor health status and disease burden.[30,32] Evidence shows that older adults were less likely to self-report poor sleep than younger individuals, especially after controlling for comorbidities and health.[33] Vitiello and colleagues[30] examined objectively measured sleep among 150 healthy older adults who reported no sleep problems and found that significant proportions of them (33% of women and 16% of men) had impaired objectively measured sleep. Healthy older adults may be prone to perceive good sleep quality.[34] In addition, older adults may expect their sleep will be less consolidated as they age, and they may accept some noticeable sleep changes as a part of normal aging owing to an adjustment of their perception of "acceptable" health with aging.[33,35]

As described, many sleep characteristics change with age in adulthood. For example, nocturnal sleep duration, sleep efficiency, slow wave sleep, and self-reported poor sleep decrease with age; in contrast, the number of awakenings, WASO, and daytime napping frequency increase with age. However, most of these changes stop at approximately 60 years of age. After that age, most sleep variables seem to remain largely unchanged within the older adult population.

AGE-RELATED CHANGES IN CIRCADIAN RHYTHMS

The circadian system regulates several human physiologic functions, including body temperature, heart rate, blood pressure, release of certain hormones, bone remodeling, sleep–wake rhythm, and rest–activity pattern.[36] It is well-documented in the literature that circadian rhythms become less robust with aging, which typically presents as an advance in circadian timing, a decrease in circadian amplitude, and a reduced ability to adjust to phase shifting (changes in the phase of circadian rhythms). The suprachiasmatic nucleus is the central endogenous circadian pacemaker that regulates 24-hour circadian rhythms. The disruption of circadian rhythms with advancing age may be associated with a progressive decline in the function of the suprachiasmatic nucleus.[37]

Phase Advance

The timing and structure of sleep are mainly regulated by the circadian system and homeostatic sleep regulation.[38] Older adults commonly experience an advance of sleep schedule to earlier hours. They tend to have sleepiness earlier in the evening and wake up earlier in the morning than desired.[36] This earlier sleep timing in older adults may be owing to the age-related phase advance in their circadian rhythm. This phase advance is seen not only in the sleep–wake cycle, but also in the body temperature rhythm, and in the timing of secretion of melatonin and cortisol,[39–41] all of which are about 1 hour advanced in older people compared with young adults.[42] **Fig. 2** compares the circadian phase between older and younger adults. However, Duffy and colleagues[43] found that the phase advance in sleep timing was greater than phase advance in other circadian clocks, which suggested that a mechanism (eg, sleep homeostasis) other than circadian phase advance alone may be involved in older adult's early sleep timing.

Reduced Amplitude in Circadian Rhythms

Aging is associated with a reduction in the amplitude of several circadian rhythms in older adults, including core body temperature, melatonin and cortisol secretion, activity, and sleep.[44–47] The age-related reduction in circadian amplitude may be related to sleep disruption in older adults.[48] It

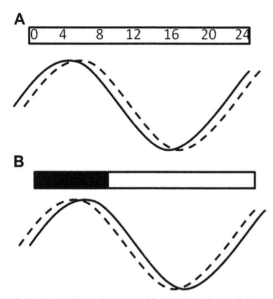

A

| 0 | 4 | 8 | 12 | 16 | 20 | 24 |

B

Fig. 2. Circadian phase in older adults. The *solid line* represents older adults' body temperature and plasma melatonin circadian profile. The *dashed line* represents young adults' body temperature and plasma melatonin circadian profile. The bar across the top of (*A*) represents the clock time. The horizontal black bar denotes the sleep or dark period. The horizontal white bar denotes wake or light period. (*A*) When compared with clock time, the phase of both core body temperature and plasma melatonin is earlier in older adults (*solid line*) than it is in young adults (*dashed line*). (*B*) When compared with their usual sleep–wake and dark–light timing, the phase of both core body temperature and plasma melatonin is later with respect to sleep/darkness in older adults (*solid line*) than it is in young adults (*dashed line*). (*From* Duffy JF, Zitting KM, Chinoy ED. Aging and circadian rhythms. Sleep Med Clin 2015;10(4):423–34).

was reported that, compared with young adults, older adults were more likely to wake up close to the timing when body temperature reached nadir.[49] This finding indicated that the biological clock (eg, body temperature) in older adults might also regulate their awakening time, which may result in even earlier awakenings in older adults.[36,49] Also, the reduced amplitude of daytime activity may result in daytime napping, which may further reduce the amplitude of the sleep–wake rhythm. Age-related decreases in the amplitude of melatonin secretion may also play a role in sleep problems in older adults[50,51] (as described elsewhere in this article).

Decreased Ability Adjusting to Phase Shifting

The ability to phase shift deceases with aging.[52] Older adults are subject to more difficulties in adjusting to phase shifts, such as shift work and

jet lag.[4,52] Monk and colleagues[53] found that older adults needed more time to recover from phase shifting, and experienced a longer period of sleep disruption and daytime disfunction. The age-related loss of rhythmic function within the suprachiasmatic nucleus may partially explain this impaired ability in phase shifting.[54]

Changes in Sleep Homeostasis

Some research indicates that the earlier sleep timing and less consolidated sleep in older adults may be attributable to the interaction between the circadian system and homeostatic regulation, rather than simply resulting from an age-related phase advance in circadian rhythm.[6,55] Sleep homeostasis regulates wake and sleep and generates sleep pressure as a function of time of being awake. Sleep pressure increases during waking and sleep deprivation, and decreases during sleep.[56] Sleep homeostasis declines with aging. The age-related decrease in TST and sleep efficiency may be partially owing to the reduced homeostatic sleep pressure with aging.[57–59] Also, this reduced homeostatic sleep pressure contributes to an increased number of nocturnal awakenings and reduced daytime sleepiness.[58,59] For example, 1 study that forced desynchronized circadian cycles found that older adults had 2.7 times more nocturnal awakenings than young individuals at most circadian phases.[10]

SLEEP-RELATED HORMONES, AGING, AND SLEEP

Age-related changes in neuroendocrine function are associated with alterations in sleep quality and sleep architecture with normal aging. We briefly review changes of several sleep-related hormones with normal aging and their associations with sleep. Most studies in this area group older adults into a single age category as compared with young or middle-aged adults, and few data exist related to hormonal changes with advancing age within the older adult age group per se.

Growth Hormone

Growth hormone (GH) secretion and slow wave sleep impact each other.[60,61] GH secretion mainly pulses during nocturnal sleep (no matter whether the sleep is advanced, delayed, or fragmented) at about 1 hour after sleep onset and decreases at transient awakenings.[62] On the other hand, the inhibition of GH-releasing hormone suppresses GH secretion, promotes corticotrophin-releasing hormone, and reduces slow wave sleep.[62,63]

Further, there is an age-related decrease in the secretion of GH.[64,65] GH secretion reaches its peak during adolescence, rapidly decreases in an exponential manner between young adulthood and middle age, and then decreases slowly between middle age and old age. This phenomenon is similar to the detected age-related decrease of slow wave sleep.[66] The decrease in nocturnal GH with aging may have a direct or indirect impact on slow wave sleep, and may be partially responsible for the observed reduction of slow wave sleep in aging.

Cortisol

Cortisol secretion has a clear circadian pattern that peaks shortly after the morning awakening, gradually declines throughout the day, and reaches its nadir in the late evening, and then increases toward the morning peak.[66] Sleep, particularly slow wave sleep, inhibits cortisol secretion.[67,68] The increase in cortisol secretion during sleep could lead to awakenings.[68,69] The circadian rhythm of cortisol changes with aging, as manifested by a decreased circadian amplitude, an increased nocturnal cortisol level, and likely a phase advanced rhythm.[63,70,71] The increased nocturnal cortisol level may contribute to decreased slow wave sleep and frequent awakenings during nocturnal sleep in older adults.[70]

Prolactin

No clear evidence shows that the secretion of prolactin affects sleep. However, sleep has an influence on prolactin secretion.[70] Sleep onset is associated with an increased secretion of prolactin, regardless of day or night sleep.[66] Also, decreased slow wave sleep or fragmented sleep may be associated with a reduced elevation of prolactin during nocturnal sleep.[66] Studies show increased prolactin secretion during slow wave sleep or by enhancing slow wave sleep, and decreased prolactin secretion in prolonged awakening during the sleep period.[72,73] Prolactin secretion during sleep may decrease with aging owing to the lighter and more fragmented sleep in older adults. Studies suggest that nocturnal prolactin in healthy older adults was significantly lower than that in young adults.[65,74]

Thyroid-Stimulating Hormone

Thyroid-stimulating hormone (TSH) secretion has a circadian pattern, which maintains a stable low level during the daytime, starts increasing in the late afternoon, peaks around sleep onset, and then gradually decreases through the night, returning to its daytime level after morning awakenings.[66,75] Studies have shown that slow wave sleep was associated with inhibited nocturnal TSH secretion, and awakenings were associated with increased nocturnal TSH secretion.[76–78] The circadian release of TSH (with regard to acrophase and nadir) is maintained with aging.[70] However, research suggests that the overall 24-hour TSH secretion is decreased in older adults.[79]

Melatonin

The 24-hour profile of plasma melatonin is primarily regulated by the light–dark circle and the sleep–wake cycle.[66] Melatonin normally remains stable at a low level during the daytime, starts to increase progressively in the evening (2 hours before habitual bedtime) and remains elevated duringthe middle of the sleep period, and then decreases gradually to its daytime level in the morning (8–9 am).[66] The onset of evening sleepiness correlates with the increase in evening melatonin secretion. Overall melatonin secretion decreases with aging, but daytime melatonin (which is already at a low basal level) may remain unchanged with aging. The increase in nocturnal melatonin in older adults was significantly reduced when compared with young adults.[50,80] Studies suggest that the age-related decreases in melatonin secretion contributes to the increased sleep disruption in older adults.[50]

Sex Hormones

Changes in gonadotropins and sex steroids with aging are associated with sleep changes in older adults. In men, testosterone levels decrease progressively with aging after 30 years of age.[81,82] Older men may also lose the diurnal testosterone pattern.[83] The decreased testosterone with aging may relate to the increased sleep fragmentation in older adults.[70] In women, estradiol levels decrease and follicle-stimulating hormone levels increase significantly during the menopause transition and after menopause. These changes in reproductive hormones have been associated with increased complaints of difficulty falling asleep and staying asleep.[70] Also, the decreased levels of endogenous estrogen and progesterone may have a negative impact on the upper airway, thereby increasing the incidence of sleep-disordered breathing after menopause.[84]

RISK FACTORS FOR SLEEP DISTURBANCES IN OLDER ADULTS

As reviewed, most sleep parameters decrease with age until the age of 60 years, but remain generally unchanged after 60 years of age. Also, older adults are less likely to complain of sleep problems and tend to accept some noticeable sleep alterations as normal changes with aging. The age-associated sleep changes discussed herein are mostly relevant to older adults who have excellent health and are aging successfully. In the real world, medical comorbidities and psychiatric illness, primary sleep disorders, and changes in social engagement, lifestyle, and environment commonly accompany aging. These factors contribute to sleep disturbances in older adults. Indeed, up to 50% to 60% of older adults reported poor sleep quality.[4,52] Therefore, sleep problems reported in older adults are usually multifactorial and are not necessarily be explained by age alone.

Medical Comorbidities and Psychiatric Illness

Approximately 67% of older adults have multiple comorbidities.[85] Osteoarthritis, cardiovascular disease, lung disease, gastroesophageal reflux, cancer, and diabetes are the most commonly reported medical comorbidities in older adults.[4,86] About 90% of adults aged 65 and older take prescription drugs to treat their chronic medical conditions. More than one-third of them routinely take more than 5 medications.[87,88] The discomfort and emotional distress from medical conditions contribute to an increased number of nocturnal awakenings and EDS in older adults. Also, chronic medical conditions are positively associated with the diagnosis or prevalence of sleep disorders, including insomnia, sleep apnea, and restless legs syndrome.[89] Of note, not only do these medical conditions cause sleep disturbances in older adults, but these sleep disturbances can also have a negative impact on medical illnesses and their associated symptoms. Evidence also shows that the multiple medications that older adults take can result in EDS, worsen primary sleep disorders, and contribute to comorbid insomnia.[89,90]

Depression and anxiety, prevalent psychiatric problems among older adults, commonly coexist with insomnia in older adults. Epidemiologic studies reported that more than 50% of older adults with depression have insomnia. Further, longitudinal studies have found that insomnia may increase the risk of depression in older adults. In addition, depression has been positively associated with EDS and the diagnosis and severity of obstructive sleep apnea.[90]

Primary Sleep Disorders

Several primary sleep disorders that are common in older adults contribute to poor sleep in older adults. These sleep disorders include insomnia, sleep-disordered breathing, periodic limb movements in sleep, restless legs syndrome, and REM sleep behavior disorder. Epidemiologic studies found that the prevalence of these primary sleep disorders is considerably higher in older adults than that in younger adults.[91,92] Medical and psychological comorbidities of aging contribute to the increased rebalance of insomnia symptoms (approximately 50%) in older adults. Interestingly, the prevalence of insomnia in older adults with excellent health is similar to that of younger adults.[93] The increase in sleep-disordered breathing frequency in older adults may partially be owing to an age-related reduction in pharyngeal muscle function and an increase in comorbidities in older adults.[94] The presentation of these primary sleep disorders contribute to poor sleep in older adults, in terms of difficulties in falling asleep, increased number of nocturnal awakenings, EDS, and complaints of nonrestorative sleep.[91]

Social, Lifestyle, and Environmental Factors

Many social and lifestyle change with aging contribute to sleep problems in older adults. Retired older adults have more flexible sleep schedules (which can be irregular), have more opportunity to nap during the day, are more sedentary, and are less involved in social activity than they used to be.[95,96] These factors affect both sleep homeostasis and circadian regulation, thus contributing to sleep disturbances. In addition, the loss of loved ones can produce emotional distress and loneliness, which are known to contribute to sleep disturbance.[4] Environmentally, many older adults, especially those who have multiple morbidities, lose independence in activities of daily living, and may move to new homes or long-term care facilities. This transition can be a major life event in later life and create several physical and psychological stressors. Sleep problems can be heightened or get worse during and after this transition. Finally, other environmental factors, such as temperature, noise, and light exposure, are also associated with sleep quality in older adults.[97,98]

SUMMARY

Sleep changes with normal aging. In general, aging is associated with advanced sleep timing, decreased nocturnal sleep time and sleep efficiency, increased frequency of daytime naps, increased nocturnal awakenings, and decreased slow wave sleep. Most sleep parameters remain unchanged after 60 years of age in healthy older adults. Circadian system and sleep homeostasis become less robust with normal aging. The amount and pattern of sleep-related hormone secretion change in normal aging. All these changes contribute to or correlate with age-related changes in sleep. Poor sleep quality and sleep disturbances are not necessarily owing to aging alone, even though sleep schedule, sleep quantity, and sleep architecture change with age. Multiple factors that accompany the aging process, including medical and psychiatric conditions, and environmental, social and lifestyle changes, can contribute to sleep problems in older adults.

REFERENCES

1. Foley D, Ancoli-Israel S, Britz P, et al. Sleep disturbances and chronic disease in older adults: results of the 2003 National Sleep Foundation Sleep in America Survey. J Psychosomatic Res 2004;56(5): 497–502.
2. Ohayon MM, Carskadon MA, Guilleminault C, et al. Meta-analysis of quantitative sleep parameters from childhood to old age in healthy individuals: developing normative sleep values across the human lifespan. Sleep 2004;27(7):1255–73.
3. Espiritu JR. Aging-related sleep changes. Clin Geriatr Med 2008;24(1):1–14, v.
4. Vitiello MV. Sleep in normal aging. Sleep Med Clin 2006;1(2):171–6.
5. Campbell SS, Murphy PJ. The nature of spontaneous sleep across adulthood. J Sleep Res 2007; 16(1):24–32.
6. Dorffner G, Vitr M, Anderer P. The effects of aging on sleep architecture in healthy subjects. Adv Exp Med Biol 2015;821:93–100.
7. Floyd JA, Janisse JJ, Jenuwine ES, et al. Changes in REM-sleep percentage over the adult lifespan. SLEEP 2007;30(7):829.
8. Floyd JA, Medler SM, Ager JW, et al. Age-related changes in initiation and maintenance of sleep: a meta-analysis. Res Nurs Health 2000;23(2):106–17.
9. Floyd JA, Janisse JJ, Marshall Medler S, et al. Nonlinear components of age-related change in sleep initiation. Nurs Res 2000;49(5):290–4.
10. Klerman EB, Davis JB, Duffy JF, et al. Older people awaken more frequently but fall back asleep at the same rate as younger people. Sleep 2004;27(4): 793–8.
11. Potari A, Ujma PP, Konrad BN, et al. Age-related changes in sleep EEG are attenuated in highly intelligent individuals. Neuroimage 2017;146:554–60.
12. Fang W, Li Z, Wu L, et al. Longer habitual afternoon napping is associated with a higher risk for impaired fasting plasma glucose and diabetes mellitus in older adults: results from the Dongfeng-Tongji cohort of retired workers. Sleep Med 2013;14(10):950–4.
13. Cao Z, Shen L, Wu J, et al. The effects of midday nap duration on the risk of hypertension in a middle-aged and older Chinese population: a preliminary evidence from the Tongji-Dongfeng cohort study, China. J Hypertens 2014;32(10): 1993–8 [discussion: 1998].
14. Furihata R, Kaneita Y, Jike M, et al. Napping and associated factors: a Japanese nationwide general population survey. Sleep Med 2016;20:72–9.
15. Milner CE, Cote KA. Benefits of napping in healthy adults: impact of nap length, time of day, age, and experience with napping. J Sleep Res 2009;18(2): 272–81.
16. Buysse DJ, Browman KE, Monk TH, et al. Napping and 24-hour sleep/wake patterns in healthy elderly and young adults. J Am Geriatr Soc 1992;40(8): 779–86.
17. Ficca G, Axelsson J, Mollicone DJ, et al. Naps, cognition and performance. Sleep Med Rev 2010; 14(4):249–58.
18. Yoon IY, Kripke DF, Youngstedt SD, et al. Actigraphy suggests age-related differences in napping and nocturnal sleep. J Sleep Res 2003;12(2):87–93.
19. Beh HC. A survey of daytime napping in an elderly Australian population. Aust J Psychol 1994;46(2): 100–6.
20. Stong KL, Ancoli-Israel S. Napping in older adults. In: Avidan AY, Alessi C, editors. Geriatric sleep medicine. 1st edition. New York: Informa Healthcare USA, Inc; 2008. p. 227–40.
21. Naska A, Oikonomou E, Trichopoulou A, et al. Siesta in healthy adults and coronary mortality in the general population. Arch Intern Med 2007;167(3):296–301.
22. Foley DJ, Vitiello MV, Bliwise DL, et al. Frequent napping is associated with excessive daytime sleepiness, depression, pain, and nocturia in older adults: findings from the National Sleep Foundation '2003 Sleep in America' Poll. Am J Geriatr Psychiatry 2007;15(4):344–50.
23. Chasens ER, Sereika SM, Weaver TE, et al. Daytime sleepiness, exercise, and physical function in older adults. J Sleep Res 2007;16(1):60–5.
24. Jaussent I, Bouyer J, Ancelin ML, et al. Excessive sleepiness is predictive of cognitive decline in the elderly. Sleep 2012;35(9):1201–7.
25. Empana JP, Dauvilliers Y, Dartigues JF, et al. Excessive daytime sleepiness is an independent risk indicator for cardiovascular mortality in community-dwelling elderly: the Three City Study. Stroke 2009; 40(4):1219–24.
26. Whitney CW, Enright PL, Newman AB, et al. Correlates of daytime sleepiness in 4578 elderly persons: the cardiovascular health study. Sleep 1998;21(1):27–36.
27. Lopes JM, Dantas FG, Medeiros JL. Excessive daytime sleepiness in the elderly: association with cardiovascular risk, obesity and depression. Rev Bras Epidemiol 2013;16(4):872–9.

28. Blachier M, Dauvilliers Y, Jaussent I, et al. Excessive daytime sleepiness and vascular events: the Three City Study. Ann Neurol 2012;71(5):661–7.

29. Bixler E, Vgontzas A, Lin HM, et al. Excessive daytime sleepiness in a general population sample: the role of sleep apnea, age, obesity, diabetes, and depression. J Clin Endocrinol Metab 2005; 90(8):4510–5.

30. Vitiello MV, Larsen LH, Moe KE. Age-related sleep change: gender and estrogen effects on the subjective-objective sleep quality relationships of healthy, noncomplaining older men and women. J Psychosom Res 2004;56(5):503–10.

31. Luo J, Zhu G, Zhao Q, et al. Prevalence and risk factors of poor sleep quality among Chinese elderly in an urban community: results from the Shanghai aging study. PLoS One 2013;8(11):e81261.

32. Foley DJ, Monjan A, Simonsick EM, et al. Incidence and remission of insomnia among elderly adults: an epidemiologic study of 6,800 persons over three years. Sleep 1999;22(Suppl 2):S366–72.

33. Gooneratne NS, Vitiello MV. Sleep in older adults: normative changes, sleep disorders, and treatment options. Clin Geriatr Med 2014;30(3):591–627.

34. Gooneratne NS, Bellamy SL, Pack F, et al. Case-control study of subjective and objective differences in sleep patterns in older adults with insomnia symptoms. J Sleep Res 2011;20(3):434–44.

35. Brouwer WB, van Exel NJ, Stolk EA. Acceptability of less than perfect health states. Soc Sci Med 2005; 60(2):237–46.

36. Wright KP, Frey DF. Age related changes in sleep and circadian physiology: from brain mechanisms to sleep behavior. In: Avidan AY, Alessi C, editors. Geriatric sleep medicine. 1st edition. New York: 2008. p. 1–18.

37. Mattis J, Sehgal A. Circadian rhythms, sleep, and disorders of aging. Trends Endocrinol Metab 2016; 27(4):192–203.

38. Schmidt C, Peigneux P, Cajochen C. Age-related changes in sleep and circadian rhythms: impact on cognitive performance and underlying neuroanatomical networks. Front Neurol 2012;3:118.

39. Kripke DF, Elliott JA, Youngstedt SD, et al. Circadian phase response curves to light in older and young women and men. J Circadian Rhythms 2007;5(1):1.

40. Kim SJ, Benloucif S, Reid KJ, et al. Phase shifting response to light in older adults. J Physiol 2014; 592(1):189–202.

41. Duffy JF, Zitting KM, Chinoy ED. Aging and circadian rhythms. Sleep Med Clin 2015;10(4):423–34.

42. Tranah GJ, Stone KL, Ancoli-Israel S. Circadian rhythms in older adults. In: Kryger MH, Roth T, Dement WC, editors. Principles and practice of sleep medicine. 6th edition. Philadelphia: Elsevier; 2017. p. 1510–5.

43. Duffy JF, Zeitzer JM, Rimmer DW, et al. Peak of circadian melatonin rhythm occurs later within the sleep of older subjects. Am J Physiol Endocrinol Metab 2002;282(2):E297–303.

44. Czeisler CA, Dumont M, Duffy JF, et al. Association of sleep-wake habits in older people with changes in output of circadian pacemaker. Lancet 1992; 340(8825):933–6.

45. Huang YL, Liu RY, Wang QS, et al. Age-associated difference in circadian sleep-wake and rest-activity rhythms. Physiol Behav 2002;76(4–5):597–603.

46. Dijk DJ, Duffy JF. Circadian regulation of human sleep and age-related changes in its timing, consolidation and EEG characteristics. Ann Med 1999; 31(2):130–40.

47. Carrier J, Monk TH, Buysse DJ, et al. Amplitude reduction of the circadian temperature and sleep rhythms in the elderly. Chronobiol Int 1996;13(5): 373–86.

48. Van Someren EJ. More than a marker: interaction between the circadian regulation of temperature and sleep, age-related changes, and treatment possibilities. Chronobiol Int 2000;17(3):313–54.

49. Duffy JF, Dijk D-J, Klerman EB, et al. Later endogenous circadian temperature nadir relative to an earlier wake time in older people. Am J Physiol 1998;275(5):R1478–87.

50. Pandi-Perumal S, Zisapel N, Srinivasan V, et al. Melatonin and sleep in aging population. Exp Gerontol 2005;40(12):911–25.

51. Kondratova AA, Kondratov RV. The circadian clock and pathology of the ageing brain. Nat Rev Neurosci 2012;13(5):325–35.

52. Bliwise DL, Scullin MK. Normal aging. In: Kryger MH, Roth T, Dement WC, editors. Principles and practice of sleep medicine. 6th edition. Philadelphia: Elsevier; 2017. p. 25–38.

53. Monk TH, Buysse DJ, Carrier J, et al. Inducing jet lag in older people: directional asymmetry. J Sleep Res 2000;9(2):101–16.

54. Farajnia S, Deboer T, Rohling JH, et al. Aging of the suprachiasmatic clock. Neuroscientist 2014;20(1): 44–55.

55. Dijk D-J, Duffy JF, Czeisler CA. Contribution of circadian physiology and sleep homeostasis to age-related changes in human sleep. Chronobiol Int 2000;17(3):285–311.

56. Taillard J, Philip P, Coste O, et al. The circadian and homeostatic modulation of sleep pressure during wakefulness differs between morning and evening chronotypes. J Sleep Res 2003;12(4):275–82.

57. Dijk DJ, Duffy JF, Riel E, et al. Ageing and the circadian and homeostatic regulation of human sleep during forced desynchrony of rest, melatonin and temperature rhythms. J Physiol 1999;516(Pt 2):611–27.

58. Carrier J, Land S, Buysse DJ, et al. The effects of age and gender on sleep EEG power spectral

density in the middle years of life (ages 20-60 years old). Psychophysiology 2001;38(2):232–42.

59. Dijk DJ, Groeger JA, Stanley N, et al. Age-related reduction in daytime sleep propensity and nocturnal slow wave sleep. Sleep 2010;33(2):211–23.

60. Gronfier C, Luthringer R, Follenius M, et al. A quantitative evaluation of the relationships between growth hormone secretion and delta wave electroencephalographic activity during normal sleep and after enrichment in delta waves. Sleep 1996;19(10):817–24.

61. Holl RW, Hartman ML, Veldhuis JD, et al. Thirty-second sampling of plasma growth hormone in man: correlation with sleep stages. J Clin Endocrinol Metab 1991;72(4):854–61.

62. Van Cauter E, Caufriez A, Kerkhofs M, et al. Sleep, awakenings, and insulin-like growth factor-I modulate the growth hormone (GH) secretory response to GH-releasing hormone. J Clin Endocrinol Metab 1992;74(6):1451–9.

63. Van Cauter E, Leproult R, Kupfer DJ. Effects of gender and age on the levels and circadian rhythmicity of plasma cortisol. J Clin Endocrinol Metab 1996;81(7):2468–73.

64. Van Cauter E, Leproult R, Plat L. Age-related changes in slow wave sleep and REM sleep and relationship with growth hormone and cortisol levels in healthy men. JAMA 2000;284(7):861–8.

65. van Coevorden A, Mockel J, Laurent E, et al. Neuroendocrine rhythms and sleep in aging men. Am J Physiol 1991;260(4 Pt 1):E651–61.

66. Copinschi G, Caufriez A. Sleep and hormonal changes in aging. Endocrinol Metab Clin North Am 2013;42(2):371–89.

67. Bierwolf C, Struve K, Marshall L, et al. Slow wave sleep drives inhibition of pituitary-adrenal secretion in humans. J Neuroendocrinol 1997;9(6):479–84.

68. Caufriez A, Moreno-Reyes R, Leproult R, et al. Immediate effects of an 8-h advance shift of the rest-activity cycle on 24-h profiles of cortisol. Am J Physiol Endocrinol Metab 2002;282(5):E1147–53.

69. Follenius M, Brandenberger G, Bandesapt JJ, et al. Nocturnal cortisol release in relation to sleep structure. Sleep 1992;15(1):21–7.

70. Buckley TM. Neuroendocrine and homeostatic changes in the elderly. In: Pandi-Perumal SR, Monti JM, Monjan AA, editors. Principles and practice of geriatric sleep medicine. 1st edition. New York: Cambridge University Press; 2010. p. 85–96.

71. Nater UM, Hoppmann CA, Scott SB. Diurnal profiles of salivary cortisol and alpha-amylase change across the adult lifespan: evidence from repeated daily life assessments. Psychoneuroendocrinology 2013;38(12):3167–71.

72. Spiegel K, Luthringer R, Follenius M, et al. Temporal relationship between prolactin secretion and slow-wave electroencephalic activity during sleep. Sleep 1995;18(7):543–8.

73. Blyton DM, Sullivan CE, Edwards N. Lactation is associated with an increase in slow-wave sleep in women. J Sleep Res 2002;11(4):297–303.

74. Greenspan SL, Klibanski A, Rowe JW, et al. Age alters pulsatile prolactin release: influence of dopaminergic inhibition. Am J Physiol 1990;258(5 Pt 1):E799–804.

75. Brabant G, Prank K, Ranft U, et al. Physiological regulation of circadian and pulsatile thyrotropin secretion in normal man and woman. J Clin Endocrinol Metab 1990;70(2):403–9.

76. Goichot B, Brandenberger G, Saini J, et al. Nocturnal plasma thyrotropin variations are related to slow-wave sleep. J Sleep Res 1992;1(3):186–90.

77. Goichot B, Buguet A, Bogui P, et al. Twenty-four-hour profiles and sleep-related variations of cortisol, thyrotropin and plasma renin activity in healthy African melanoids. Eur J Appl Physiol Occup Physiol 1995;70(3):220–5.

78. Hirschfeld U, Moreno-Reyes R, Akseki E, et al. Progressive elevation of plasma thyrotropin during adaptation to simulated jet lag: effects of treatment with bright light or zolpidem. J Clin Endocrinol Metab 1996;81(9):3270–7.

79. Van Coevorden A, Laurent E, Decoster C, et al. Decreased basal and stimulated thyrotropin secretion in healthy elderly men. J Clin Endocrinol Metab 1989;69(1):177–85.

80. Zeitzer JM, Duffy JF, Lockley SW, et al. Plasma melatonin rhythms in young and older humans during sleep, sleep deprivation, and wake. Sleep 2007;30(11):1437–43.

81. Shi Z, Araujo AB, Martin S, et al. Longitudinal changes in testosterone over five years in community-dwelling men. J Clin Endocrinol Metab 2013;98(8):3289–97.

82. Harman SM, Metter EJ, Tobin JD, et al, Baltimore Longitudinal Study of Aging. Longitudinal effects of aging on serum total and free testosterone levels in healthy men. Baltimore Longitudinal Study of Aging. J Clin Endocrinol Metab 2001;86(2):724–31.

83. Bremner WJ, Vitiello MV, Prinz PN. Loss of circadian rhythmicity in blood testosterone levels with aging in normal men. J Clin Endocrinol Metab 1983;56(6):1278–81.

84. Lin CM, Davidson TM, Ancoli-Israel S. Gender differences in obstructive sleep apnea and treatment implications. Sleep Med Rev 2008;12(6):481–96.

85. Salive ME. Multimorbidity in older adults. Epidemiol Rev 2013;35:75–83.

86. Fillenbaum GG, Pieper CF, Cohen HJ, et al. Comorbidity of five chronic health conditions in elderly community residents: determinants and impact on mortality. J Gerontol A Biol Sci Med Sci 2000;55(2):M84–9.

87. Kaufman DW, Kelly JP, Rosenberg L, et al. Recent patterns of medication use in the ambulatory adult population of the United States: the Slone survey. JAMA 2002;287(3):337–44.

88. Linjakumpu T, Hartikainen S, Klaukka T, et al. Use of medications and polypharmacy are increasing among the elderly. J Clin Epidemiol 2002;55(8): 809–17.

89. Barczi SR. Sleep and medical comorbidities. In: Avidan AY, Alessi C, editors. Geriatric sleep medicine. 1st edition. New York: 2008. p. 19–36.

90. Boockvar KS. Reducing sedative-hypnotic medication use in older adults with sleep problems. Clin Ther 2016;38(11):2330–1.

91. Crowley K. Sleep and sleep disorders in older adults. Neuropsychol Rev 2011;21(1):41–53.

92. Rissling M, Ancoli-Israel S. Sleep in aging. In: Stickgold R, Walker MP, editors. Neuroscience of sleep. London, United Kingdom: Academic Press; 2009. p. 78–84.

93. Ohayon MM. Prevalence of DSM-IV diagnostic criteria of insomnia: distinguishing insomnia related to mental disorders from sleep disorders. J Psychiatr Res 1997;31(3):333–46.

94. McMillan A, Morrell MJ. Sleep disordered breathing at the extremes of age: the elderly. Breathe (Sheff) 2016;12(1):50–60.

95. Li J, Yang B, Varrasse M, et al. Sleep among long-term care residents in China a narrative review of literature. Clin Nurs Res 2016 [pii: 1054773816673175].

96. Zantinge EM, van den Berg M, Smit HA, et al. Retirement and a healthy lifestyle: opportunity or pitfall? a narrative review of the literature. Eur J Public Health 2014;24(3):433–9.

97. Li J, Grandner AM, Chang YP, et al. Person-centered dementia care and sleep in assisted living residents with dementia: a pilot study. Behav Sleep Med 2017; 15(2):97–113.

98. Hanford N, Figueiro M. Light therapy and Alzheimer's disease and related dementia: past, present, and future. J Alzheimer's Dis 2013;33(4): 913–22.

Insomnia in the Older Adult

Glenna S. Brewster, PhD, RN, FNP-BC[a,b],*, Barbara Riegel, PhD, RN[c],
Philip R. Gehrman, PhD, CBSM[b,d]

KEYWORDS

- Sleep-onset latency • Sleep efficiency • Benzodiazepines • Sleep diary • Pharmacotherapy
- Cognitive-behavioral therapy for insomnia (CBTi) • Wake after sleep onset

KEY POINTS

- The incidence of insomnia increases with aging. Insomnia can include difficulty falling asleep at the start of the sleep period, waking up during the night and having difficulty falling back asleep, and waking up early and being unable to get back to sleep. Difficulty staying asleep and early morning insomnia are common in older adults with insomnia disorder.
- When diagnosing insomnia, health care providers need to collect a thorough health history and include questions about the older adult's sleep, medical, and psychiatric history.
- Cognitive-behavioral therapy for insomnia, which consists of stimulus control, sleep restriction, sleep hygiene, and cognitive therapy, is the recommended first-line therapy for treatment of insomnia in older adults.
- Because of the higher risk for adverse effects in older patients, medications should be used sparingly and, when possible, be discontinued.
- Cognitive-behavioral therapy for insomnia has been shown to be more efficacious than medications for the long-term management of insomnia in older adults.

INTRODUCTION

Prevalence and Diagnosis of Insomnia

Sleep changes with aging. Specifically, babies sleep between 10 and 14 hours per day, whereas the recommended sleep duration for older adults is between 7 and 8 hours daily.[1] Many older adults experience dissatisfaction with the quantity and quality of sleep even with an adequate opportunity to sleep; when this is accompanied by daytime impairment over a period of time, they may meet the criteria for insomnia disorder (**Table 1**).

Compared with younger adults, the prevalence of insomnia is higher in middle and older adults[2,3] and increases with age. Up to 50% of older adults report insomnia symptoms; however, this does not mean that insomnia is a normal part of aging.[4]

Sleep onset or initial insomnia is manifested by difficulty falling asleep that occurs at the start of the sleep period.[5–7] Sleep maintenance or middle insomnia involves multiple and prolonged awakenings during the night.[5–7] Late insomnia or early morning awakenings is waking up early on mornings and being unable to return to sleep.[5–7] Older adults

Disclosure Statement: The authors have no financial or commercial disclosures. G.S. Brewster is a Ruth L. Kirschstein NRSA Postdoctoral Research Fellow (NIH: T32HL07713; PI: Pack, A.).
[a] Nell Hodgson Woodruff School of Nursing, Emory University, 1520 Clifton Road, Room 344, Atlanta, GA 30322, USA; [b] Center for Sleep and Circadian Neurobiology, Perelman School of Medicine of the University of Pennsylvania, 3624 Market Street, Suite 201, Philadelphia, PA 19104, USA; [c] School of Nursing, University of Pennsylvania, Room 418 Curie Boulevard, 335 Fagin Hall, Philadelphia, PA 19104, USA; [d] Department of Psychiatry, Perelman School of Medicine of the University of Pennsylvania, 3535 Market Street, Suite 670, Philadelphia, PA 19104, USA
* Corresponding author.
E-mail address: glenna.brewster@emory.edu

Sleep Med Clin 13 (2018) 13–19
https://doi.org/10.1016/j.jsmc.2017.09.002
1556-407X/18/

Table 1
Diagnostic criteria for insomnia

Diagnostic Criteria for Chronic Insomnia (*ICSD-3*)[44]	Diagnostic Criteria for Chronic Insomnia (*DSM-5*)[5]

Criteria A–F must be met:
A. Patients report, or patients' parent or caregiver observes, one or more of the following:
  1. Difficulty initiating sleep
  2. Difficulty maintaining sleep
  3. Waking up earlier than desired
  4. Resistance to going to bed on appropriate schedule
  5. Difficulty sleeping without parent or caregiver intervention
B. Patients report, or the patients' parent or caregiver observes, one or more of the following related to the nighttime sleep difficulty:
  1. Fatigue/malaise
  2. Attention, concentration, or memory impairment
  3. Impaired social, family, occupational, or academic performance
  4. Mood disturbance/irritability
  5. Daytime sleepiness
  6. Behavioral problems (eg, hyperactivity, impulsivity, aggression)
  7. Reduced motivation/energy/initiative
  8. Proneness for errors/accidents
  9. Concerns about or dissatisfaction with sleep
C. The reported sleep/wake complaints cannot be explained purely by inadequate opportunity (ie, enough time is allotted for sleep) or inadequate circumstances (ie, the environment is safe, dark, quiet, and comfortable) for sleep.
D. The sleep disturbance and associated daytime symptoms occur at least 3 times per week.
E. The sleep disturbance and associated daytime symptoms have been present for at least 3 mo.
F. The sleep/wake difficulty is not explained more clearly by another sleep disorder.
	A. There is a predominant complaint of dissatisfaction with sleep quantity or quality, associated with one (or more) of the following symptoms:
	  1. Difficulty initiating sleep (In children, this may manifest as difficulty initiating sleep without caregiver intervention.)
	  2. Difficulty maintaining sleep, characterized by frequent awakenings or problems returning to sleep after awakenings. (In children, this may manifest as difficulty returning to sleep without caregiver intervention.)
	  3. Early morning awakening with inability to return to sleep
	B. The sleep disturbance causes clinically significant distress or impairment in social, occupational, educational, academic, behavioral, or other important areas of functioning.
	C. The sleep difficulty occurs at least 3 nights per week.
	D. The sleep difficulty is present for at least 3 mo.
	E. The sleep difficulty occurs despite adequate opportunity for sleep.
	F. The insomnia is not better explained by and does not occur exclusively during the course of another sleep-wake disorder (eg, narcolepsy, a breathing-related sleep disorder, a circadian rhythm sleep-wake disorder, a parasomnia).
	G. The insomnia is not attributable to the physiologic effects of a substance (eg, a drug of abuse, a medication).
	H. Coexisting mental disorders and medical conditions do not adequately explain the predominant complaint of insomnia.
	Specify if
	• *Episodic:* symptoms last at least 1 mo but <3 mo
	• *Persistent:* symptoms last 3 mo or longer
	• *Recurrent:* 2 (or more) episodes within the space of 1 y

Abbreviations: DSM-5, Diagnostic and Statistical Manual of Mental Disorders (Fifth Edition); ICSD-3, International Classification of Sleep Disorders, Third Edition.

tend to have more challenges with sleep maintenance compared with younger adults,[3,4,8] which results in reductions in total sleep time and sleep efficiency.[8] Insomnia can also be situational, persistent, or recurrent.[5] Situational insomnia is usually acute insomnia that lasts a few days or weeks and is associated with changes in the sleep schedule or the sleep environment.[5,8] Life events, such as retirement, hospitalizations, and new-onset illnesses, can precipitate situational insomnia.

Usually when the event that triggers the insomnia is resolved, so too does the insomnia. If the insomnia does not resolve, it evolves into chronic insomnia.[5] Recurrent insomnia is episodic and often returns with the occurrence of stressful life events.[5]

Risk Factors of Insomnia

Multiple factors increase the risk for older adults developing insomnia. They include environmental, behavioral, medical, and social factors[8] (**Table 2**). For example, older adults may change their usual bedtime and wake time after they retire increasing their risk for developing insomnia. Also, older adults also tend to have more comorbid disorders and are using multiple medications, which further increases their risk for sleep disturbances.[2,3]

EVALUATION OF INSOMNIA

Insomnia is diagnosed through a detailed clinical history taken from patients and their bed partner.[9] In order to diagnose the specific type of insomnia, it is important for clinicians to ask about the history of insomnia, insomnia symptoms, sleep-wake routines and patterns, other sleep-related symptoms, daytime functioning and consequences, and previous treatments.[9,10] Older adults should also be asked about whether they snore or have leg discomfort.[11] Clinicians need to also identify whether there are comorbid medical, substance, and/or psychiatric conditions impacting sleep.[10] Suggested screening tests for psychiatric disorders that can be used include: the Patient Health Questionnaire-9,[12] the Geriatric Depression Scale,[13] and the General Anxiety Disorder Questionnaire.[14] It is also important to assess daytime activities, as older adults may be less active during the day and consequently spend more time napping or dozing.

Subjective measures that can be used to evaluate sleep include sleep patterns questionnaires, like the Pittsburgh Sleep Quality Index (PSQI) and the Insomnia Severity Index (ISI), and sleep diaries. The PSQI is a 19-item instrument that assesses sleep quality and disturbances over a 1-month interval.[15] Scores can range between 0 and 21, with a score of 5 or more suggestive of poor sleep quality.[15] The ISI is a 7-item questionnaire that assesses the nighttime symptoms and impact of insomnia over the previous month.[16] Scores range from 0 to 28, with values greater than 14 suggestive of moderate to severe insomnia.[16]

Sleep diaries allow for the prospective tracking of an individual's sleep/wake patterns. They capture information like bedtime, time to fall asleep, number and duration of nightly awakenings, wake-up time, out-of-bed time, and times and duration of daytime naps or dozing.[9,17] Sleep diaries may also include questions about sleep quality, and types and amounts of medications, caffeine, and alcohol consumed.[9] Sleep diaries completed for approximately 2 weeks allows for the recognition of sleep patterns and variability.[9] Older patients sometime have difficulties completing sleep diaries because of visual impairments. Large print can be used for the sleep diaries given to these older adults to enhance the ease of completion of the diaries.

Table 2 Risk factors for insomnia in older adults	
Environment	Excessive noise, hot or cold temperatures, light during the sleep period Moving to a new home or downsizing to a smaller space or a retirement community or related facility Institutionalization
Behavioral/social	Irregular sleep schedules, caffeine use later in the day, alcohol close to bedtime Caregiving, hospitalizations, new medical problems Retirement or lifestyle change Death of a family member or friend Inappropriate use of social drugs, for example, alcohol (Note that alcohol is frequently used to self-medicate for sleep problems. It helps with falling asleep; however, when the effect wears off, sleep becomes light and disrupted.) Napping
Demographics	Female sex
Medical	Medications: theophylline, thyroid hormone, anticholinergics, stimulants, oral decongestants, antidepressants, corticosteroids, antihypertensives, opioids, nonsteroidal antiinflammatory drugs Sleep disorders: sleep apnea, restless leg syndrome, periodic limb movement disorder, rapid eye movement disorder, age-related circadian rhythm change (phase advance) Psychiatric and cognitive conditions: depression, anxiety, mania, panic attacks, schizophrenia, substance abuse, dementia Other medical conditions: diabetes, fibromyalgia, hypertension, cardiovascular disease, stroke, chronic pain

Data from Refs.[2,5,8,9,34]

Objective assessments of sleep, such as actigraphy and polysomnography, are not necessary for routine diagnosis and assessment of insomnia; but they may be helpful to rule out other comorbid sleep disorders, such as sleep-disordered breathing or circadian rhythm sleep-wake disorders.[18–20]

TREATMENTS FOR INSOMNIA

The goal of insomnia treatment is the improvement of sleep quality and/or quantity, and reduction in insomnia-related daytime impairments.[9] Patients should be involved in the development of the treatment plan and decisions about which treatment goals to pursue because buy-in from patients is critical for success.[21] The choice of treatment depends on the severity and duration of the insomnia symptoms, coexisting disorders, willingness of patients to engage in behavioral therapies, and vulnerability of patients to the adverse effects of medications.[9] It is important to emphasize to patients that it is normal to have occasional nights of poor sleep during and after the completion of treatment so that they will have realistic expectations about treatment and cope better during treatment.[21]

Sleep diaries and questionnaires can be used to evaluate how the treatment is progressing and to determine when there has been sufficient improvement to warrant discontinuation of treatment.[9] After treatment is discontinued, it is important to conduct periodic follow-ups to identify potential recurrence and precipitating events due to changes in health or lifestyle.

Nonpharmacologic Treatment Options

Cognitive-behavioral therapy for insomnia (CBTi) is a multicomponent intervention involving cognitive and behavioral techniques like stimulus control therapy, sleep restriction therapy, relaxation training, cognitive restructuring, and sleep hygiene education.[22] The goal of CBTi is to replace maladaptive thoughts and sleep habits and to reduce arousal associated with sleep.[22] CBTi has produced both short-term and long-term improvement in sleep.[23] Although CBTi is effective for insomnia, many health care providers are neither aware of the existence of CBTi nor know how to refer patients for treatment.[24]

- Stimulus control aims to strengthen the association between the bed/bedroom and sleep and to produce a consistent sleep-wake schedule. Instructions for stimulus control include minimize napping; go to bed only when sleepy; get out of bed if unable to sleep; use the bed/bedroom only for sleep and sex; and wake up at the same time each day.[22]
- Sleep restriction is used to increase the homeostatic drive for sleep in order to improve sleep quality. The time spent in bed is reduced to the actual sleep duration based on sleep diaries, which creates some mild sleep deprivation. The time in bed is then gradually increased until the individual achieves an optimal sleep duration.[22] There is strong support for sleep restriction in older adults with insomnia.[25] Sleep compression is an alternative technique to sleep restriction whereby time in bed is gradually reduced until the older adult achieves an optimal sleep duration.[26]
- Relaxation training is done to reduce tension and intrusive thoughts that interfere with the ability to sleep. The relaxation techniques used include deep-breathing exercises, progressive muscle relaxation, biofeedback, and guided imagery.[22]
- Cognitive restructuring aims to reduce worry and change misconceptions associated with sleep and insomnia using Socratic questioning.[22] Challenging inaccurate patterns of thinking can change how older adults perceive the effect of sleep on their lives.
- Sleep hygiene education provides some guidelines about factors that may help or interfere with sleep. They include not eating a heavy meal or drinking alcohol within 2 hours of bedtime; limiting caffeine intake after lunchtime; exercising regularly but not within 2 hours of bedtime; and keeping the bedroom quiet, dark, and at a cool, comfortable temperature.[22]

Mindfulness-based stress reduction techniques aim to change reactions to stress by teaching purposeful awareness and acceptance of the present state[27] and includes techniques, such as breathing, body scan, walking meditations, and Hatha yoga.[28] These techniques have been effective in reducing insomnia in older adults.[28]

Bright light therapy helps to strengthen circadian rhythms and establish a healthy sleep-wake cycle.[29,30] The results have been mixed on its efficacy for the treatment of insomnia in older adults[29,30] but in general may have a favorable effect when used with older adults.[29] Health care practitioners can recommend white light sources with a bluish tint that provides at least 1000 lux at the eye during daytime hours; at a time that is most convenient for patients; on mornings after awakening if the circadian timing of patients is unknown; or during the time interval patients tend to be more tired.[29]

Acupuncture is a traditional Chinese technique in which specific points on the body are stimulated, usually by inserting thin needles through the skin.[31] It has been shown to be effective in improving insomnia symptoms in older adults.[31]

Pharmacologic Treatment Options

Benzodiazepines, such as lorazepam, temazepam, and clonazepam, decrease sleep latency and nocturnal awakenings; they also reduce rapid eye movement (REM) sleep.[32] In older adults, they increase the risk for memory impairment, falls, fractures, motor vehicle accidents, and avoidable emergency department visits and hospital admissions; therefore, their use should be avoided in older adults.[33,34] Between 5.3% and 10.8% of adults aged 50 years and older use benzodiazepines.[35] Long-term use of benzodiazepines can promote psychological dependence, and there is an increased risk of addiction and abuse.[36] Tolerance can also develop over time, thus, requiring larger doses to sustain the efficacy.[36] It is necessary to educate older adults about the effects of benzodiazepine use and encourage discontinuation through tapering.[33,37] Although there is no current standard for tapering benzodiazepines, some providers recommend establishing a longer tapering schedule over 4 to 5 months for older patients and tapering the dose by 25% every 2 weeks.[33,37,38] While tapering, health care providers could provide CBTi.[37,38]

Nonbenzodiazepine hypnotics reduce sleep latency.[32] These medications, which include eszopiclone, zolpidem, and zaleplon, should be avoided in older adults without consideration of the duration of use (no more than 90 days) because they can cause confusion and they increase the risk of falls and fractures. These medications should be avoided in older adults with dementia and cognitive impairment.[34]

Melatonin receptor agonists reduce sleep latency and increase sleep duration.[1,39] An example is ramelteon. The potential adverse effects include mild gastrointestinal disturbances and nervous system effects, such as dizziness, headache, somnolence, and fatigue, with no evidence of significant rebound insomnia or withdrawal effects.[39]

Many *antidepressants* have sedating effects and are sometimes used to treat insomnia, often at lower doses than used for depression. Antidepressants often have overall REM-suppressing effects and can decrease slow-wave sleep latency and the duration of slow-wave sleep.[32] In the absence of an underlying depressive disorder, antidepressants should also be avoided in older adults because they are highly anticholinergic, are sedating, increase the risk of falls, and cause orthostatic hypotension.[34]

Antihistamines decrease sleep latency;[32] however, these over-the-counter sleep medications, like diphenhydramine, produce rapid tolerance and are highly anticholinergic.[34] Anticholinergic effects include blurred vision, dizziness, difficulty urinating, dry mouth, and constipation. Anticholinergic medications can also increase the risk for cognitive impairment and decline; therefore, drugs with a high anticholinergic profile, such as antihistamines, should be avoided in older adults.[34]

Melatonin and valerian root are classified as complementary and alternative medications. They are supplements and are not regulated by the Food and Drug Administration. The doses and the preparations available to consumers usually vary significantly. Melatonin is an endogenous hormone secreted by the pineal gland but is also used as an exogenous supplement.[40,41] Melatonin decreases subjective sleep latency in some studies, although it may cause headaches and drowsiness.[40,41] Valerian root has been shown to improve subjective sleep parameters, but the research is less consistent with objective sleep parameters. Rare side effects reported for valerian root include gastrointestinal upset, contact allergies, headache, and restless sleep.[40] Individuals using complementary and alternative medications should always inform their health care provider and consider the interactions between herbal remedies and prescription medications.[40]

Pharmacologic treatments should only be used for the short-term management of insomnia. When pharmacotherapy is used, health care providers should consider the insomnia symptoms, whether other treatments are available, how patients responded to previous treatments, the side effect profile of the medication, and medication interactions.[36] Older adults have better response rates with lower dosages because decreased lean body mass, increased body fat, and reduction in plasma proteins may increase blood concentration of unbound drugs and the drug half-life.[36] Therefore, when prescribing medications for insomnia for older adults, start with the lowest dose and titrate upward.[36] Given the side effects and concerns about the long-term safety, it is recommended that pharmacotherapy for insomnia be avoided or be used only for short periods of time.[34,42]

Comparative Effectiveness of Cognitive-Behavioral Therapy for Insomnia and Medications

A comparative effectiveness study of CBTi compared with sleep medications (zopiclone, zolpidem, temazepam, or triazolam) found that CBTi is as effective for the short-term treatment of insomnia as medications.[24,43] The effects of CBTi may also be more long-lasting than medications.[22,24] Although medications produce more rapid improvements compared with CBTi, over the long-term, CBTi has more durable and sustained effects on sleep quality and outcomes. The therapeutic effects of medications are usually not maintained after the medication is discontinued.[24]

SUMMARY

Aging is associated with several changes in sleep continuity and architecture parameters. Many older adults experience difficulties with falling asleep, staying asleep, or waking up too early, which leads to daytime impairment and warrants a diagnosis of insomnia. Factors, such as the sleep environment, medications, and medical and psychiatric disorders, can increase the risk for insomnia. Therefore, health care providers should obtain a comprehensive health and sleep history from older adults in order to correctly diagnose insomnia and identify the potential correlates of the disorder. After diagnosing insomnia, the first-line treatment is CBTi. Medications, such as benzodiazepines and nonbenzodiazepines, should be avoided in older adults given their potential for significant adverse consequences and clinical guidelines recommending against their use.

REFERENCES

1. Hirshkowitz M, Whiton K, Albert SM, et al. National Sleep Foundation's sleep time duration recommendations: methodology and results summary. Sleep Health 2015;1(1):40–3.
2. Blay SL, Andreoli SB, Gastal FL. Prevalence of self-reported sleep disturbance among older adults and the association of disturbed sleep with service demand and medical conditions. Int Psychogeriatrics 2008;20(3):582–95.
3. Leblanc MF, Desjardins S, Desgagné A. Sleep problems in anxious and depressive older adults. Psychol Res Behav Management 2015;8:161–9.
4. Ohayon MM. Epidemiology of insomnia: what we know and what we still need to learn. Sleep Med Rev 2002;6(2):97–111.
5. American Psychiatric Association. Sleep-wake disorders. In: Diagnostic and statistical manual of mental disorders. 5th edition. Arlington (VA): American Psychiatric Publishing; 2013.
6. Lichstein KL, Durrence HH, Taylor DJ, et al. Quantitative criteria for insomnia. Behav Res Ther 2003; 41(4):427–45.
7. Lineberger MD, Carney CE, Edinger JD, et al. Defining insomnia: quantitative criteria for insomnia severity and frequency. Sleep 2006;29(4):479–85.
8. Vitiello MV. Sleep in normal aging. Sleep Med Clin 2012;7(3):539–44.
9. Schutte-Rodin S, Broch L, Buysse D, et al. Clinical guideline for the evaluation and management of chronic insomnia in adults. J Clin Sleep Med 2008; 4(5):487–504.
10. Mai E, Buysse DJ. Insomnia: prevalence, impact, pathogenesis, differential diagnosis, and evaluation. Sleep Med Clin 2008;3(2):167–74.
11. McCall WV. Sleep in the elderly: burden, diagnosis, and treatment. Prim Care Companion J Clin Psychiatry 2004;6(1):9–20.
12. Kroenke K, Spitzer RL, Williams JBW. The PHQ-9: validity of a brief depression severity measure. J Gen Intern Med 2001;16(9):606–13.
13. Yesavage JA, Brink TL, Rose TL, et al. Development and validation of a geriatric depression screening scale: a preliminary report. J Psychiatr Res 1982; 17(1):37–49.
14. Wild B, Eckl A, Herzog W, et al. Assessing generalized anxiety disorder in elderly people using the GAD-7 and GAD-2 scales: results of a validation study. Am J Geriatr Psychiatry 2014;22(10): 1029–38.
15. Buysse DJ, Reynolds CF 3rd, Monk TH, et al. The Pittsburgh Sleep Quality Index: a new instrument for psychiatric practice and research. Psychiatry Res 1989;28(2):193–213.
16. Bastien CH, Vallieres A, Morin CM. Validation of the insomnia severity index as an outcome measure for insomnia research. Sleep Med 2001;2(4):297–307.
17. Carney CE, Buysse DJ, Ancoli-Israel S, et al. The consensus sleep diary: standardizing prospective sleep self-monitoring. Sleep 2012;35(2):287–302.
18. Littner M, Hirshkowitz M, Kramer M, et al. Practice parameters for using polysomnography to evaluate insomnia: an update. Sleep 2003;26(6):754–60.
19. Ancoli-Israel S, Cole R, Alessi C, et al. The role of actigraphy in the study of sleep and circadian rhythms. Sleep 2003;26(3):342–92.
20. Roehrs T. Sleep physiology and pathophysiology. Clin Cornerstone 2000;2(5):1–15.
21. Gooneratne NS, Vitiello MV. Sleep in older adults: normative changes, sleep disorders, and treatment options. Clin Geriatr Med 2014;30(3):591–627.
22. Morin CM, Bootzin RR, Buysse DJ, et al. Psychological and behavioral treatment of insomnia: update of the recent evidence (1998-2004). Sleep 2006; 29(11):1398–414.

23. Alessi C, Martin JL, Fiorentino L, et al. Cognitive behavioral therapy for insomnia in older veterans using nonclinician sleep coaches: randomized controlled trial. J Am Geriatr Soc 2016;64(9):1830–8.

24. Mitchell MD, Gehrman P, Perlis M, et al. Comparative effectiveness of cognitive behavioral therapy for insomnia: a systematic review. BMC Fam Pract 2012;13:40.

25. McCurry SM, Logsdon RG, Teri L, et al. Evidence-based psychological treatments for insomnia in older adults. Psychol Aging 2007;22(1):18–27.

26. Lichstein KL, Riedel BW, Wilson NM, et al. Relaxation and sleep compression for late-life insomnia: a placebo-controlled trial. J Consulting Clin Psychol 2001;69(2):227–39.

27. Ong JC, Manber R, Segal Z, et al. A randomized controlled trial of mindfulness meditation for chronic insomnia. Sleep 2014;37(9):1553–63.

28. Zhang JX, Liu XH, Xie XH, et al. Mindfulness-based stress reduction for chronic insomnia in adults older than 75 years: a randomized, controlled, single-blind clinical trial. Explore (NY) 2015;11(3):180–5.

29. Sloane PD, Figueiro M, Cohen L. Light as therapy for sleep disorders and depression in older adults. Clin Geriatr 2008;16(3):25–31.

30. Gammack JK. Light therapy for insomnia in older adults. Clin Geriatr Med 2008;24(1):139–49, viii.

31. Kwok T, Leung PC, Wing YK, et al. The effectiveness of acupuncture on the sleep quality of elderly with dementia: a within-subjects trial. Clin Interv Aging 2013;8:923–9.

32. Pagel JF, Parnes BL. Medications for the treatment of sleep disorders: an overview. Prim Care Companion J Clin Psychiatry 2001;3(3):118–25.

33. Tannenbaum C. Inappropriate benzodiazepine use in elderly patients and its reduction. J Psychiatry Neurosci 2015;40(3):E27–8.

34. By the American Geriatrics Society Beers Criteria Update Expert Panel. American Geriatrics Society 2015 updated beers criteria for potentially inappropriate medication use in older adults. J Am Geriatr Soc 2015;63(11):2227–46.

35. Olfson M, King M, Schoenbaum M. Benzodiazepine use in the United States. JAMA Psychiatry 2015; 72(2):136–42.

36. Kamel NS, Gammack JK. Insomnia in the elderly: cause, approach, and treatment. Am J Med 2006; 119(6):463–9.

37. Bélanger L, Belleville G, Morin C. Management of hypnotic discontinuation in chronic insomnia. Sleep Med Clin 2009;4(4):583–92.

38. Paquin AM, Zimmerman K, Rudolph JL. Risk versus risk: a review of benzodiazepine reduction in older adults. Expert Opin Drug Saf 2014;13(7):919–34.

39. Roth T, Seiden D, Sainati S, et al. Effects of ramelteon on patient-reported sleep latency in older adults with chronic insomnia. Sleep Med 2006;7(4): 312–8.

40. Gooneratne NS. Complementary and alternative medicine for sleep disturbances in older adults. Clin Geriatr Med 2008;24(1):121–38, viii.

41. Buscemi N, Vandermeer B, Hooton N, et al. The efficacy and safety of exogenous melatonin for primary sleep disorders: a meta-analysis. J Gen Intern Med 2005;20(12):1151–8.

42. Perlis M, Gehrman P, Riemann D. Intermittent and long-term use of sedative hypnotics. Curr Pharm Des 2008;14(32):3456–65.

43. Sivertsen B, Omvik S, Pallesen S, et al. Cognitive behavioral therapy vs zopiclone for treatment of chronic primary insomnia in older adults: a randomized controlled trial. JAMA 2006;295(24):2851–8.

44. American Academy of Sleep Medicine. International classification of sleep disorders. 3rd edition. Darien (IL): American Academy of Sleep Medicine; 2014.

Apnea in Older Adults

Susmita Chowdhuri, MD, MS[a,b,*], Pragnesh Patel, MD[b],
M. Safwan Badr, MD[a,b]

KEYWORDS

- Aging • Sleep • Cardiovascular • Hypertension • Stroke • Cognitive • Quality of life • CPAP

KEY POINTS

- Epidemiologic studies indicate that sleep-disordered breathing (SDB), including central sleep apnea, has a higher prevalence in the older adult population compared with younger and middle-aged adults. The underlying pathophysiology for this increased prevalence remains unresolved.
- Evolving research reveals that SDB in older adults is linked to an increased risk for stroke, heart failure, atrial fibrillation, type 2 diabetes, excessive daytime sleepiness, and early cognitive decline.
- There is conflicting evidence regarding the risk for mortality and for developing incident hypertension and ischemic heart disease; moreover there is a paucity of evidence regarding SDB effects on driving accidents and quality of life in older adults.
- The impact of positive airway pressure therapy on clinical outcomes in older adults is not well studied.
- There are no systematic outcome data on the impact of alternative therapies, including oral appliances and bariatric surgery, in older adults with SDB.

INTRODUCTION

Sleep disordered breathing (SDB) is more prevalent in older adults than in young and middle-aged adults. By 2050, 1 in 5 people will be 60 years or older prompting the World Health Organization to adopt a global 5-year strategy and action plan for enhancing older adult health (2016–2020) to alleviate complications of chronic diseases.[1] Given the very high prevalence of a chronic diseases like SDB in the United States and Europe, it is imperative that health care agencies focus on SDB and alleviate its adverse consequences in older adults to ensure that older adults live longer and healthier lives. The following sections review the current evidence and highlight research gaps related to the diagnosis and management of SDB in older adults.

EPIDEMIOLOGY

Several large, community-based epidemiologic studies have demonstrated increased prevalence of SDB in people older than 60 years of age, ranging from 27% to 80%.[2–6] Ancoli-Israel and colleagues[3] estimated the prevalence of SDB was 27% in community-dwelling older adults and 42% in nursing home residents. A population-based study in healthy adults noted that 3%, 33%, and 39% of 60, 70, and 80 year olds, respectively,[4] had an apnea-hypopnea index (AHI) of 5 or greater, with predominantly central apneas. Additionally, the prevalence of obstructive sleep apnea (OSA) (AHI ≥5) in the age group older than 71 years was 80% and increased 2.2 fold for each 10 years of advancing age.[6] Men are twice as likely to have SDB as women.[4,6] The prevalence of central apnea

Conflict of Interest: None.
[a] Sleep Medicine Section, John D. Dingell VA Medical Center, Detroit, MI 48201, USA; [b] Department of Medicine, Wayne State University, Detroit, MI 48201, USA
* Corresponding author. Medical Service, John D. Dingell VA Medical Center, 4646 John R (11M), Detroit, MI 48201.
E-mail address: schowdh@med.wayne.edu

(defined as a central apnea index [CAI] of ≥ 2.5) increased from 1.7% in the middle-aged group to 12.1% in the older-age group (odds ratio [OR] = 8.3).[5] The age-specific prevalence of a CAI of 20 or greater for men older than 65 years was 5.2%. However, the prevalence of a CAI greater than 0 in women was only 0.3%.[7] In the Outcomes of Sleep Disorders in Older Men (MrOS) sleep study, a study of community-based sample of older men, the prevalence of moderate-severe SDB using an AHI cutoff of 15 was 21.4% to 26.4%,[8] that is, higher than in younger adults.[9] This prevalence was similar to the prevalence in older adults of the Sleep Heart Health Study (SHHS)[10] and in a subgroup of men aged 65 years and older from a Pennsylvania-based cohort.[5] The AHI increases over time with longitudinal follow-up; older heavier adults have the highest rate of increase in AHI over time.[11,12]

In summary, the available studies indicate a higher prevalence of SDB in older adults, particularly men, relative to middle-aged adults, with a noted increase in the prevalence of central apneas.

CLINICAL MANIFESTATIONS

The main symptoms of SDB in older adults are snoring and excessive daytime sleepiness (EDS).[13,14] In the community-based MrOS sleep study, older men had a 50% greater odds of sleepiness if they had SDB.[8] However, in a separate study, only 32% of older individuals had EDS with Epworth sleepiness scale (ESS) scores greater than 10[15]; however, ESS may underestimate EDS in older adults. Moreover, some older adults may underestimate daytime napping. In one study, 40% of individuals who fell asleep at least twice during a multiple sleep latency test (MSLT) did not perceive their naps and had lower Modified Mini-Mental State Examination (MMSE) scores than matched individuals who perceived their naps.[16]

Older patients with SDB may also present with insomnia. In a study of older veterans undergoing behavioral therapy for insomnia, nearly half had occult SDB, which was characterized by reported EDS but not snoring or witnessed breathing pauses.[17] Significant predictors for SDB in the MrOS sleep study were age, obesity, Asian versus Caucasian race, snoring, sleepiness, hypertension, cardiovascular (CV) disease, and heart failure.[8]

The association of SDB with body mass index (BMI) is weaker in older versus middle-aged individuals.[18] But in one study, BMI more accurately identified the presence of a mild form of OSA, whereas male sex and central fat distribution better defined the presence of severe cases in older adults.[19]

DIAGNOSTIC TESTING

Attended full nocturnal polysomnography (PSG) remains the gold standard for diagnosing SDB in older adults. Older patients receiving home care services who had multiple comorbid conditions and a high pretest probability on the Berlin questionnaire were more likely to have a diagnosis of OSA.[20] Limited channel study recording in the sleep laboratory was reliable when compared with in-laboratory PSG in older patients.[21] Moreover, in-home unattended home sleep apnea testing (HSAT) that recorded airflow combined with symptoms of sleep apnea, BMI, neck circumference, age, and sex, was the best-performing 2-stage model for the diagnosis of OSA in older adults with an area under the curve (AUC) of 0.85 and negative posttest probability of 0.5% to make a diagnosis of OSA defined as an AHI of 30 or greater.[22]

In summary, population- and clinic-based studies suggest that the prevalence of snoring and EDS is high in older individuals with SDB. The ESS and sleep questionnaires have not been validated in older adults. The home sleep testing pathway needs to be further delineated in older adults.

PATHOPHYSIOLOGY

Sleep state oscillations may precipitate central apnea and periodicity in older adults (**Fig. 1**).[23,24] Pack and colleagues noted a waxing and waning oscillatory breathing pattern during the lighter stages of sleep in older subjects suggesting that ventilatory control mechanisms were involved.[23,24] The authors' group has demonstrated that healthy (nonapneic) older adults have narrower carbon dioxide (CO_2) reserve than younger adults because of the high controller gain,[25] but this was not noted in older patients with OSA.[26] The effects of aging on chemo-responsiveness during *wakefulness* have also yielded conflicting results.[27,28] During sleep, there was no change in the magnitude of the hypercapnic ventilatory response.[29] In contrast, Chowdhuri and colleagues[30] demonstrated that during non–rapid eye movement (*NREM*) *sleep*, older adults had an increased isocapnic hypoxic ventilatory response and hyperoxic suppression of ventilation (Dejours' effect) despite the absence of ventilatory long-term facilitation (plasticity) following acute intermittent hypoxia. Additionally, cerebral blood flow (CBF) regulation and cerebrovascular responsiveness to CO_2 (CVR) are reduced in older adults that may also reduce the CO_2 reserve.[31,32] Thus, increased chemosensitivity, unconstrained by respiratory plasticity and reduced CVR, may explain

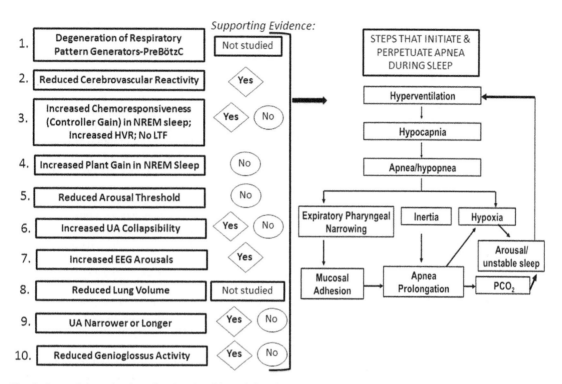

Fig. 1. Potential mechanisms for SDB in older adults. This image depicts the potential underlying pathophysiologic mechanisms that may contribute to increased SDB in the elderly and the limited or conflicting evidence in humans to support these (*left panel*). See text for more discussion of the evidence. The panel on the right provides an overview of the pathways that lead to the development and perpetuation of apnea/hypopnea during sleep in humans. The image demonstrates the potential underlying pathophysiologic mechanisms that may contribute to increased SDB in older adults (*left panel*) and the limited or conflicting evidence in humans to support these. mechanisms. See text for a detailed description. An overview of the mechanisms leading to apnea/hypopnea during sleep (*right panel*) is also presented; specifically, a transient increase in minute ventilation will result in increased alveolar Po_2 and decreased Pco_2 and a subsequent ventilatory response, opposite to the initial perturbation. The central apnea may initiate several processes, including inertia of the ventilatory control system, hypoxia, and transient arousal; moreover, central apnea is associated with upper airway narrowing and/or occlusion upper airway obstruction may occur when the ventilatory drive reaches a nadir during induced periodic breathing. The development of upper airway obstruction during central apnea, combined with mucosal and gravitational factors, delays pharyngeal opening, often requiring a transient arousal to restore respiration, which may perpetuate breathing instability. HVR, hypoxic ventilatory response; LTF, long-term facilitation of ventilation; NREM, non–rapid eye movement; PreBötC, pre-Bötzinger complex; UA, upper airway.

the increased propensity for central apneas in older individuals during sleep. Additionally, because ablation of the pre-Bötzinger complex (pre-BötC) in animal models resulted in apnea,[33] it is postulated that degeneration of pre-BötC neurons may contribute to central sleep apnea (CSA) in older adults.

Although some studies showed narrowed upper airway (UA) dimensions and collapsibility in older versus young adults, others have not.[34–36] There was no effect of aging on the arousal threshold[36] or genioglossus (GG) electromyographic activity.[37] Conversely, the GG response to hypoxia was reduced.[38] The length of the airway, an important determinant of airway stability, was not greater in older versus young adults.[35] Edwards and colleagues[39] found that older patients with OSA had a more collapsible airway and a lower loop gain; however, the study was restricted to participants with OSA and not designed to test the effect of aging per se on the underlying traits.

In summary, there are inconclusive data regarding the relative contributions of central breathing instability versus UA anatomy to the development of SDB in older adults.

CONSEQUENCES OF SLEEP-DISORDERED BREATHING IN OLDER ADULTS

Severe SDB (AHI ≥30) is associated with significant adverse CV health consequences in middle-aged individuals. Although there has been controversy about whether SDB has health consequences in older adults,[40,41] recent studies indicate a significant increased health risk of SDB in older adults (**Tables 1** and **2**).

Hypertension

Whether SDB increases the risk of hypertension in older adults remains uncertain given the conflicting findings in the literature. Cross-sectional analysis of the SHHS showed that SDB was not associated with systemic hypertension in those aged 60 years or older.[42] Whether this was a consequence of survival bias or if smaller blood pressure (BP) and heart rate responses to arousal in older adults is protective[43] is uncertain. Conversely, a French study reported that an AHI of 30 or greater was independently associated with incident hypertension, after 3 years, in normotensive older adults ($P = .02$; OR 1.8; 95% confidence interval [CI] 1.1–2.8).[44] Older adult normotensive patients with SDB were also at risk for having masked daytime hypertension and nighttime nondipping of BP. However, in a cohort of older community-dwelling men, the AHI, level of hypoxemia, sleep duration, and arousal index were not independently associated with an increased risk of hypertension.[45]

In summary, cross-sectional and longitudinal studies provide conflicting results about whether SDB in older adults is associated with hypertension or not.

Cardiovascular Events

Early studies noted conflicting CV consequences of SDB in older adults. Whereas studies in younger adults showed that an AHI of 5 or greater significantly increased the risk of CV events and death,[46,47] older adults did not have an increase in cardiac events, ischemic heart disease (IHD), or mortality even with severe OSA.[48–50] A large, multiethnic, community-based study noted that an increasing AHI category and hypoxia were significantly associated with an increased left ventricular mass in individuals aged 65 years or younger but not in those aged greater than 65 years.[51] The authors speculated that there may be age variations in the susceptibility to CVD, such as, magnitude of inspiratory effort generated with each apneic event, patterns of apneas across the night, and autonomic responses to apneas, which may be less pronounced in individuals older than 65 years leading to survival bias.

In contrast, several clinic-based observational studies have reported an increased mortality in older patients with moderate to severe OSA as well as a protective effect from continuous positive airway pressure (CPAP) treatment. Older patients with severe OSA (AHI ≥30) had shorter survival compared with mild OSA (AHI <15), even after adjusting for sex, BMI, AHI, and pulmonary and cardiac diseases.[52] A study in Spain that followed 939 older patients (aged ≥65 years) with OSA over 69 months demonstrated that untreated, severe OSA was associated with an increase in the risk of all-cause mortality, death from stroke, and death from heart failure; but there was no association with an increased risk of death from IHD compared with the control group.[53] AHI as a continuous variable was independently associated with increased CV mortality (hazard ratio [HR] 1.01, 95% CI 1.00–1.02); specifically, untreated severe OSA was associated with death from stroke and heart failure, but not with death from coronary heart disease. The discrepancy between the SHHS and the Spanish study results may be explained by the fact that, whereas the SHHS was population based, the Spanish sample was clinic based, with a high percentage of patients with severe OSA (62.6%) and a prior history of CV events (38.5%).

Moreover, in a longitudinal study over 13.8 years, EDS (MSLT) and self-reported sleep parameters were associated with an increased all-cause mortality risk in older adults with SDB[54] and the risk was even higher with EDS combined with an AHI of 20 or greater and persisted after adjusting for covariates, including sleep duration greater than 8.5 hours, self-reported angina, male sex, African American race, and age.

Heart failure is also associated with an increased prevalence of SDB. The association of AHI with heart failure was similar in men older than and younger than 70 years, (adjusted HR 1.58, 95% confidence interval (CI) 0.93–2.66) for those with an AHI of 30 or greater compared with those with an AHI less than 5.[49] Additionally, in a community-based cohort of older men,[55] having central apneas (CAI ≥5) and the presence of Cheyne-Stokes respiration (CSR), but not obstructive AHI, were significant predictors of incident heart failure. After excluding those with baseline heart failure, the incident risk of heart failure was attenuated for those with a CAI of 5 or greater but remained significantly elevated for those with CSR.

Cross-sectional analysis of the MrOS sleep study data (n = 2911 participants, aged ≥65 years), using a single-lead electrocardiogram examination, revealed that the increasing severity of SDB was associated with increased odds of nocturnal atrial fibrillation (AF) and complex ventricular ectopy (CVE),[56] and incident AF over a 6.5-year period was predicted by CSA (OR 2.58; 95% CI 1.18–5.66) and CSR with CSA (OR 2.27, 95% CI 1.13–4.56) but not by OSA or hypoxemia.[57] In individuals greater than 76 years of

Table 1
Results from studies of cardiovascular events, mortality, stroke, and diabetes in older adults

Author	Study and Sample Characteristics	Age Mean ± SD or Range (y)	Results
HTN			
Prospective studies			
Guillot et al,[44] 2013	Population-based cohort, 372 normotensive subjects; follow-up 3 y	68.0 ± 1.1	An AHI of ≥30 is associated with an increased risk of incident HTN (OR 1.77, 95% CI 1.11–2.80).
Fung et al,[45] 2011	Population-based, 243 with criteria for incident hypertension; follow-up 3.4 y	75.1 ± 4.9	The SWS percentage was significantly associated with incident HTN (OR for lowest to highest quartile of SWS 1.83, 95% CI 1.18–2.85).
Cross-sectional studies			
Endeshaw et al,[96] 2009	Community-dwelling, 70 participants, 57% women	74.9 ±6.4	Moderate to severe SDB (AHI ≥15) increased the risk for nocturnal HTN (P = .03) with significantly lower BP dipping during sleep; AHI significantly predicted increased night-day systolic BP ratio (β = .002, t = 2.959, P = .004).
Haas et al,[42] 2005	Population-based, cross-sectional analysis of the Sleep Heart Health Study, 6120 participants	Stratified by age: 40–59 y vs >60 y (70.2 ± 6.9)	In those aged <60 y, AHI was significantly associated with higher odds of systolic/diastolic HTN (AHI 15.0–29.9, OR = 2.38, 95% CI 1.30–4.38; AHI ≥30, OR = 2.24, 95% CI 1.10–4.54). Among those aged ≥60 y, no association between AHI and systolic/diastolic HTN was found. Isolated systolic HTN was not associated with SDB in either age category.
Cardiac Events and Mortality			
Prospective studies			
Ancoli-Israel et al,[52] 2003	Inpatient ward, 350 men; follow-up 5.7 ± 4.5 y	69 ± 7	There were significantly greater mortality rates in patients who had both CHF and CSA vs just CHF or just CSA or just OSA; for those with CHF, having CSA shortened the life span (HR 1.66, P = .012); having OSA had no effect. Age was a significant predictor of CHF (coefficient 0.0127, P = .028).

(continued on next page)

Table 1
(continued)

Author	Study and Sample Characteristics	Age Mean ± SD or Range (y)	Results
Mant et al,[97] 1995	Local population, 163 participants, follow-up 4 y	84	SDB with RDI ≥15 was not a predictor of mortality (OR 0.99, CI 0.94–1.04).
Gottlieb et al,[49] 2010	Community-based population, 4422 subjects (56% women) free of CHD and heart failure at baseline; median follow-up 8.7 y	58–74 with AHI ≥30	AHI associated with heart failure was similar in men older and younger than 70 y (adjusted HR for incident heart failure of 1.58, 95% CI 0.93–2.66) for those with AHI ≥30 vs AHI <5.0. OSA predicted incident heart failure in men but not in women, (adjusted HR 1.13, 95% CI 1.02–1.26 per 10-unit increase in AHI). OSA predicted incident coronary heart disease only in men aged <70 y (adjusted HR 1.68 for those with AHI ≥30 vs AHI <5).
Tuohy et al,[50] 2016	Medicare fee-for-service registry of patients initiating dialysis over a 6-y period, 184,217 patients	72–82	SDB was associated with slightly lower risks of death (HR 0.93, 95% CI 0.91– 0.96), myocardial infarction (HR 0.92, 95% CI 0.87–0.98), and ischemic stroke (HR 0.90, 95% CI 0.82–0.98) and was not associated with AF (HR 1.02, CI 0.98–1.07).
Martinez-Garcia et al,[98] 2009	Patients admitted for stroke, 166 patients with ischemic stroke, 59% men; follow-up 5 y	73.3 ± 11	Patients with SDB AHI ≥20 who did not tolerate CPAP had an increased adjusted risk of mortality (HR 2.69, 95% CI 1.32–5.61) compared with AHI <20, and an increased adjusted risk of mortality (HR 1.58, 95% CI 1.01–2.49; P<.04) compared with patients with moderate to severe OSA who tolerated CPAP.
Martinez-García et al,[53] 2012	Clinic-based population, 939 participants, 60%–70% men; median follow-up 69 mo	71.9 ± 4.5 (severe OSA)	Compared with the control group, untreated severe OSA was associated with an increase in the risk of all-cause mortality (HR 1.99, 95% CI 1.42–2.81; P = .001) from stroke (HR 4.63, 95% CI 1.03–20.8; P = .046) and from heart failure (HR 3.93, 95% CI 1.13–13.65; P = .031); but there was no association with an increased risk of death from IHD (HR 1.09, 95% CI 0.37–3.36; P = .23). The mortality risk was low for the CPAP-treated group (HR 0.93, 95% CI 0.46–1.89); there was no increase in mortality risk for the untreated mild- moderate OSA group (HR 1.38, 95% CI 0.73–2.64). CPAP compliance as a continuous variable was independently associated with a lower risk of CV mortality (HR 0.48, 95% CI 0.30–0.78; P = .003).

Study	Description	Age	Findings
Gooneratne et al,[54] 2011	Community-based, 289 participants, 71.9% women; follow-up of 13.8 y	78.0 ± 6.3	SDB (AHI ≥20) with excessive daytime sleepiness was associated with increased mortality (adjusted mortality HR 2.3, 95% CI 1.5–3.6), adjusted for sleep duration >8.5 h, self-reported angina, male sex, African American race, and age.
Johansson et al,[99] 2012	Community-based, 331 participants; follow-up 7 y	Mean 78	Compared with those with no SDB and OSA, more participants with CSA had a left ventricular EF <50%, IHD, and TIA/stroke. Longitudinal follow-up: CSA (not OSA) was a risk for all-cause mortality (HR 1.7, $P = .027$) but not for CV mortality (HR 1.7, $P = .17$).
Munoz et al,[59] 2006	394 initially event-free subjects without CPAP, 57.1% men; mean follow-up 4.5 y	Median 77.3	20 ischemic strokes were registered. Severe OSA, AHI ≥30 at baseline, had an increased risk of developing a stroke (adjusted HR 2.52, 95% CI 1.04–6.01, $P = .04$).
Stone et al,[58] 2015	Community-based study, 2872 men; mean follow-up 7.3 y	76.34 ± 5.51	Severe nocturnal hypoxemia (≥10% of the night with Spo_2 levels less than 90%) had an increased risk of incident stroke compared with those without nocturnal hypoxemia (relative adjusted HR 1.83, 95% CI 1.12–2.98; P trend = .02); nocturnal hypoxemia was also associated with a significant 2.8–3.2-fold increase in risk for fatal stroke.
Javaheri et al,[55] 2016	Community-based, 2865 men; mean follow-up 7.3 ± 2.2 y	76.3 ± 5.5	The presence of CAI ≥5 (adjusted HR 1.79, 95% CI 1.16–2.77) and presence of Cheyne-Stokes breathing (adjusted HR, 2.23, 95% CI 1.45–3.43) but not obstructive AHI were significant predictors of incident heart failure; the risk remained significantly elevated for those with Cheyne-Stokes breathing (HR 1.90, 95% CI 1.10–3.30) even after excluding patients with baseline heart failure.
May et al,[57] 2016	Community-based study, 843 men without prevalent atrial fibrillation; mean follow-up 6.5 ± 0.7 y	75 ± 5	CSA was associated with incident AF (OR 2.58, 95% CI 1.18–5.66) and so was Cheyne-Stokes respiration with CSA (OR 2.27, 95% CI 1.13–4.56); but OSA or hypoxemia did not predict incident AF. AF was related to central apnea (OR, 9.97, 95% CI 2.72–36.50), Cheyne-Stokes respiration with central apnea (OR 6.31, 95% CI 1.94–20.51), and AHI (OR 1.22, 95% CI 1.08–1.39 [per 5-unit increase]).

(continued on next page)

Table 1
(continued)

Author	Study and Sample Characteristics	Age Mean ± SD or Range (y)	Results
Holmqvist et al,[100] 2015	A national outcomes registry for AF, 10,132 participants; follow-up 2 y	75 (67–82)	Physician-defined OSA had a higher risk of hospitalization (HR 1.12, 95% CI 1.03–1.22; P = .0078) but no difference in the risks of CV death (HR 0.94, 95% CI 0.77–1.15; P = .54), composite of CV death, myocardial infarction, and stroke/TIA (HR 1.07, 95% CI 0.85–1.34; P = .57) or AF progression (HR 1.06, 95% CI 0.89–1.28; P = .51). Patients with OSA on CPAP treatment were less likely to progress to more permanent forms of AF compared with patients without CPAP (HR 0.66, 95% CI 0.46–0.94; P = .021)
Cross-sectional studies			
Javaheri et al,[51] 2016	Community-based study, 1412 participants; 46.4% men	68 ± 8.8	The left ventricular mass was significantly increased with increasing AHI category for those aged 65 y or younger (β = 1.84 ± 0.47 g/m, P = .0001) and not for older-age adults.
Mehra et al,[56] 2009	Community-based study, 2911 men	76.4 ± 5.5	There were 138 participants with AF (4.7%) and 1048 with CVE (36.0%). After adjusting for potential confounders, including HF, an association was noted between CSR-CSA and AF (OR 4.54, 95% CI 2.96–6.96). An increasing RDI quartile was associated with increased odds of CVE. The highest RDI quartile was associated with increased odds of CVE (fully adjusted OR 1.37, 95% CI 1.08–1.75). CSA was more strongly associated with AF (OR 2.69, 95% CI 1.61–4.47) than CVE (OR 1.27, 95% CI 0.97–1.66). The hypoxia level was associated with CVE (P value for trend, <.001).
Type 2 Diabetes Mellitus			
Strand et al,[40] 2015	Community-based prospective study, 5888 participants; mean follow-up 5.1 y	73.6 ± 5.8 with EDS	Incident type 2 diabetes was positively associated with observed apnea (HR 1.84, 95% CI 1.19–2.86), snoring (HR 1.27, 95% CI 0.95–1.71), and daytime sleepiness (HR 1.54, 95% CI 1.13–2.12).

Abbreviations: AF, atrial fibrillation; AHI, apnea-hypopnea index; BP, blood pressure; β, beta coefficient; CHF, congestive heart failure; CI, confidence interval; CPAP, continuous positive airway pressure therapy; CSA-CSR, central sleep apnea with Cheyne-Stokes Respiration; CV, cardiovascular; CVE, complex ventricular ectopy; EF, ejection fraction; HR, hazard ratio; HTN, hypertension; IHD, ischemic heart disease; RDI, respiratory disturbance index; Sao_2, oxygen saturation; SD, standard deviation; SWS, slow wave sleep; TIA, transient ischemic attack.

age, incident AF was related to both central and obstructive events.

In summary, a small number of clinic-based longitudinal studies indicate there is an increased all-cause and CV mortality risk attributable to severe OSA in the older adult population, whereas general population-based studies suggest the contrary. The incidence of IHD was not increased, but the risk for incident heart failure and AF was high in older patients with CSA with CSR.

Cerebrovascular Disease

In the MrOS sleep study, 5.4% of older men with SDB had a stroke over a period of 7.3 years of follow-up.[58] After adjustment for age, clinic site, race, BMI, and smoking status, older men with severe nocturnal hypoxemia had a 1.8-fold increased risk of incident stroke compared with those without nocturnal hypoxemia. Increased stroke was also seen in patients with severe OSA in a clinic-based study.[59]

In summary, results from 2 prospective observational studies suggest that there is an increased risk for stroke in older adults with SDB, independent of other risk factors. The underlying mechanisms remain unknown.

Excessive Daytime Sleepiness and Cognitive Function

Frequent oxygen desaturation (oxygen desaturation index ≥15 events) and percentage of sleep time in apnea or hypopnea (>7%) are associated with developing mild cognitive impairment (MCI) and dementia, but sleep fragmentation and sleep duration is not.[60] Cognitive impairment in patients with sleep apnea seems to be age dependent.[61,62] Older adults with milder SDB (AHI 10–20) may have cognitive dysfunction only in the presence of excessive sleepiness.[63] In a cross-sectional sample of healthy older individuals, daytime sleepiness was found in only 9.2% of patients[64] and no significant association was found between AHI, nocturnal hypoxemia, and cognitive scores. But older women with SDB were more likely to develop MCI or dementia than those without SDB.[60] Alchanatis and colleagues[62] demonstrated that cognitive deterioration in patients with SDB was age dependent, and aging patients (aged >50 years) were less able to compensate for the cognitive consequences of SDB. In the MrOS sleep study, the oxygen desaturation index and the percentage of sleep time with oxygen saturation less than 90% were associated with subsequent decline in global cognitive function.[65] An 8-year longitudinal population-based study of 559 healthy older subjects (60% women) found that SDB was associated with a significant decline in attention and memory that was more evident in the group with an AHI greater than 30, even after controlling for multiple comorbidities.[66] This finding may be due to sleep fragmentation not nocturnal hypoxemia.[67] Additionally, in older women with SDB, there was a significant association of an AHI greater than 30, and oxygen saturation nadir less than 80% with cognitive impairment. SDB also correlated with the presence of apolipoprotein E4 (ApoE4).[68] Severe SDB (AHI ≥30) was linked to measures of delayed recall and executive function in cognitively healthy older adults.[69] No significant differences were observed in physical strength, cognitive function, apathy scale, depression scale, or activities of daily living between mild to moderate OSA and severe OSA in older adults.[70]

White matter hyperintensities that indicate dementia have been linked to SDB in older adults.[71] Increased levels of hypoxemia correlate with increased volume and thickness of gray matter of the brain[72]; potentially, chronic intermittent hypoxia from SDB may upregulate cerebral amyloid plaque formation and tau phosphorylation causing memory deficit and neuronal degeneration and axonal dysfunction[73] in older individuals with SDB.

Depression
Cross-sectional analysis of the Multi-Ethnic Study of Atherosclerosis sleep study with 1784 middle-aged and older adults found that an AHI greater than 15 as well as subjective and objective measures of sleep duration were consistently associated with higher rates of depression.[74] A case control study in older adults also found a significant association between SDB and depression.[75] Moreover, older adults with CV disease and SDB were at risk for developing sickness behavior (including reporting fatigue, difficulty initiating or maintaining sleep, pain) and depressive symptoms.[76] Women were 5.44 times more likely to have depression.[77–79]

In summary, SBD in older adults is associated with EDS, cognitive decline, and depression. It is unclear whether specific neurocognitive domains are at greater risk for impairment in older adults.

Type 2 Diabetes

The US Cardiovascular Health Study in older adults reported that symptoms of observed apnea, snoring, and daytime sleepiness were associated with higher fasting glucose levels, higher 2-hour glucose levels, and lower insulin sensitivity; when followed over 6 years, the risk of incident type 2 diabetes was related to symptoms of OSA.[39]

Table 2
Results from studies of cognitive function, mood, and functional status in older adults with sleep-disordered breathing

Author	Study and Sample Characteristics	Age Mean ± SD (y)	Results
Cognitive function and Sleepiness			
Prospective studies			
Blackwell et al,[65] 2015	Community dwelling; 2636 men (without mild cognitive impairment) Follow-up: 3.4 ± 0.5 y	76.0 ± 5.3	Men with ≥1% of sleep time with SaO_2 <90% had an adjusted annualized decline of 0.43 points on MMSE compared with 0.25 for controls (P = .003). For each 5-point increase in ODI, there was an average annualized decline of 0.36 points (P = .01). There was no association between AHI values and cognitive decline.
Yaffe et al,[60] 2011	Community-based cohort, 303 women Median follow-up: 4.7 y	82.3 ± 3.2	Elevated ODI (≥15 events/h) and a high percentage (>7%) of sleep time in apnea or hypopnea were associated with the risk of developing mild cognitive impairment (adjusted OR 1.71, 95% CI 1.04–2.83) and dementia (adjusted OR 2.04; 95% CI 1.10 – 3.78). The arousal index and total sleep time were not associated with the severity of SDB.
Lim et al,[101] 2013	Community-based cohort, 737 participants Follow-up: 3.3 ± 1.7 y	81.6 ± 7.2	A higher level of sleep fragmentation was associated with an increased risk of Alzheimer dementia (HR 1.22, 95% CI 1.03–1.44; P = .02).
Martin et al,[67] 2016	Population based, 559 participants (60% women) Follow-up: 8 y	66.9 ± 0.9	SDB was associated with a slight but significant decline in the attention domain (P = .01), more evident in the subjects with an AHI >30 (P = .004).
Cross-sectional studies			
Ju et al,[69] 2012	63 participants without cognitive disorders, 41% women	68.2 ± 4.8	Patients with severe SDB (AHI ≥30) had significant delayed recall (P = .003) and errors on the TMT part B (P = .009); ODI (β = −0.37, P = .003) and educational level (β = 0.24, P = .04) determined delayed recall impairment (adjusted coefficient of determination, R^2 = 17.8%; P = .003). TMT B errors were independently associated with educational level (β = −0.41, P = .001) and AHI (β = 0.31, P = .007; adjusted R^2 = 25.7%, P = .001).
Sforza et al,[64] 2010	Community based, 827 participants	68 ± 1.8	SDB (AHI >5) was not associated with cognitive scores; 9.2% of patients had daytime sleepiness; patients with AHI >30 had delayed recall and abnormal Stroop test.
Spira et al,[68] 2008	Community based, 448 women	82.8 ± 3.4	Cognitive impairment was noted with AHI ≥30 (OR 3.4, 95% CI 1.4–8.1) and oxygen saturation <80% (OR 2.7, 95% CI 1.1–6.6) there was an increased risk in those with ApoE4 allele.

Depression

Cross-sectional studies

Study	Sample	Age	Findings
Alcántara et al,[74] 2015	Community dwelling, 1784 participants	68.21 ± 9.09 (54–93)	AHI >15 + EDS was associated with depression in age- and site-adjusted models (adjusted prevalence ratio = 1.55, 95% CI 1.05–2.46).
Farajzadeh et al,[75] 2016	Case control study, 350 participants	Case group 69.42 ± 7.95 Control group 68.08 ± 7.48	A significant association was found between OSA and depression (OR 6.61, 95% CI 1.01–2.39).
Johansson et al,[76] 2015	Community dwelling, 331 participants, 49% men	78 ± 3	SDB-related hypoxia was associated with inflammation (β >0.40), sickness behavior (β = 0.19), and depressive symptoms (β = 0.11).
Sforza et al,[77] 2002	Sleep laboratory patients, 60 participants	50.6 ±1.6	Anxiety was present in 16% and depression in 7% cases with SDB. The HAD-D score was related to the ESS score, R = 0.37; P = .003; the ESS score alone explained the 17% of variance in the HAD-D score.
Sforza et al,[78] 2016	Population based, 825 participants, 59% female	68.8 ± 1.0	Anxiety was present in 38% of the sample and depression in 8% of sample. No differences in patients with SDB from controls in depression scores and medication intake. Women were 5.44 times more likely to have depression with a low contribution of the time with SaO2 <90%.

Functional Status and Quality of Life

Study	Sample	Age	Findings
Spira et al,[80] 2014	Prospective cohort, 302 women Follow-up: IADL and mobility measures after 5.0 ± 0.7 y	82.3 ± 3.2	Patients with AHI ≥15 had a greater risk for IADL difficulties (OR 2.22, 95% CI 1.09–4.53) and of incident IADL difficulty (OR 2.43, 95% CI 1.00–5.92). There was no association with sleep fragmentation or sleep duration.
Stepnowsky et al,[83] 2000	70 African Americans	73.6 ± 6.4	OSA was significantly related to both general physical functioning and general mental health functioning in those with mild apnea (AHI <15) but not in those with moderate to severe apnea; the quality of life remained low in moderate to severe OSA.
Martínez-García et al,[84] 2009	212 patients with AHI >10, (109>65 y, 103≤65 y)	Older age group: 66–83	In patients >65 y, the presence of OSA or excessive daytime sleepiness had no significant impact on SF-36, whereas the quality of life was reduced in younger patients.

Abbreviations: AF, atrial fibrillation; AHI, apnea-hypopnea index; CI, confidence interval; ESS, Epworth Sleep Scale; HAD-D, Hospital anxiety and depression scale; HR, hazard ratio; IADL, instrumental activities of daily living; MMSE, Mini-Mental State Examination; ODI, oxygen desaturation index; OR, odds ratio; Sao₂, oxygen saturation; SDB, sleep disordered breathing; SF-36, 36-Item Short Form Health Survey; TMT B, trail making test-part B.

Function and Quality of Life

Older women (aged 82.3 ± 3.2 years) with an AHI of 15 or greater at baseline had a greater number of instrumental activities of daily living (IADL) difficulties and incident IADL difficulty compared with normal controls,[80] after adjustment for comorbid conditions. There was no association between AHI and mobility difficulty. However, in a separate study, an AHI of 10 or greater was associated with greater ADL impairment among older adults undergoing rehabilitation following a stroke.[81] In older adults with OSA, health care costs were 2 times higher than controls and 1.93 times as high as for middle-aged patients with OSA.[82] CV disease and the use of psychoactive drugs were the independent determinants of the "most-costly" older patients with OSA.

The 36-Item Short Form Health Survey was also reduced in older African American men with OSA of any severity.[83] Conversely, in subjects older than 65 years, the presence of OSA or EDS had only a slight impact on health-related quality of life (HRQOL), relative to normal values; the principal determinants of HRQOL were the presence of comorbidities, age, oxygen desaturation parameters, and the use of psychotropic medications.[84]

Thus, there are very limited data on the effect of SDB in older adults on functional status and HRQOL.

THERAPY
Positive Airway Pressure Therapy

CPAP remains the first-line therapy for SDB therapy. Older patients may require lower CPAP levels compared with the young. It is unclear if this was related to a positive airway pressure (PAP)–induced greater decrease in airway resistance in older adults.[85] It is not known whether older adults with cognitive impairment are able to use CPAP independently. Studies demonstrate that patients with mild to moderate Alzheimer disease (AD) and with Parkinson disease wore CPAP for 4.8 and 5.2 hours per night, respectively.[86,87] However, patients with AD with depressive symptoms had worse adherence. Age was not an independent predictor of compliance with CPAP in one study. However, female sex, BMI, sleepiness, an AHI of 30 or less, and CPAP setting predicted PAP noncompliance.[88] Other predictors were cigarette smoking, nocturia, and benign prostatic hypertrophy.[89] Aloia and colleagues[90] studied the impact of intervention with two 45-minute education sessions on PAP adherence in older adults. There were no significant differences in adherence

between the therapy and control groups at weeks 1 or 4, but after 12 weeks the experimental group used CPAP 3.2 hours longer with a large effect achieved.[90]

There are no randomized controlled studies of the impact of PAP therapy on CV outcomes in older adults. In observational studies, CPAP provided protection against both fatal and nonfatal CV events in middle-aged men[91] and women.[92] CPAP therapy was associated with reduced risk of all-cause and CV mortality as well as death from stroke and heart failure to levels similar to those of patients without OSA.[53] Moreover, adherence to PAP was independently associated with a lower risk of CV mortality. A reduction of CV mortality risk or longer survival with CPAP was also observed in patients aged 75 years or older.[53,93]

CPAP may improve sleepiness but only partly reverse cognitive impairment. ESS scores were reduced in patients with AD with SDB from 8.89 during baseline to 6.56 and 5.53 after 3 and 6 weeks of CPAP treatment, respectively, but not in the sham group.[87] Moreover, continued (open-label) CPAP use (mean 13.3 months) in mild to moderate AD with SDB was associated with the stabilization of depressive symptoms, less cognitive decline and daytime somnolence, with significantly improved subjective sleep quality. Caregivers of CPAP therapy patients also reported that their sleep had improved. In a 12-month, multicenter, CPAP versus best supportive care (BSC) parallel-group randomized trial across the United Kingdom, older patients who were randomized to CPAP had improved outcomes.[94] The effect was greater in patients with higher CPAP usage or higher baseline ESS. CPAP improved objective sleepiness, mobility, total cholesterol, and LDL cholesterol at 3 months; but these were not sustained at 12 months; plus, there was no change in mood, functionality, nocturia, accidents, cognitive function, and CV events. CPAP was slightly more cost-effective than BSC.

Finally, there are no data on the efficacy or effectiveness of oral appliances (OAs) in older adults.

Oral appliance

There are no outcomes studies with OAs in older adults. In a postal survey, only 36% of older adult patients perceived the regular use of OA therapy to be effective in managing OSA.[95]

In summary, PAP therapy may improve daytime sleepiness in older adults; but the effects on cognition, function, and CV events/mortality need further elucidation.

> **Box 1**
> **Future directions for research on sleep-disordered breathing in older adults**
>
> 1. Studies to that validate the use of the Epworth sleepiness scale and other commonly used sleep questionnaires in older adults are needed.
> 2. Future studies need to determine whether HSAT has similar accuracy in older adults as in younger adults and whether there are any safety or usability considerations.
> 3. Detailed systematic experiments during NREM sleep in older adults are needed to clarify the relative contributions of ventilatory control versus upper airway anatomy towards the development of SDB in older adults.
> 4. Data from longitudinal studies with similar demographic characteristics could be pooled to clarify whether SDB in older adults increases the risk for incident or uncontrolled hypertension and CV mortality.
> 5. The determinants of incident heart failure, stroke, and arrhythmias in older patients with SDB and the impact of therapy need to be studied with longitudinal, observational, and/or randomized controlled trials.
> 6. Experimental methods should be standardized with regard to the use of neurocognitive tests that study different neurocognitive domains to determine whether older patients with SDB are at risk for early dementia.
> 7. The mechanisms and genetic underpinnings of accelerated cognitive decline in older patients with SDB need to be explored so that novel therapies can be developed to target these mechanisms.
> 8. Studies should clarify the effect of SDB on quality of life, function, and health care utilization in older adults.
> 9. Randomized controlled studies with PAP, OA, and bariatric surgery are required to determine the impact of intervention on CV, metabolic, and neurocognitive outcomes.
> 10. Given that CSA is common in older adults, the impact of therapy with auto-PAP needs to be studied further.

SUMMARY

SDB has a high prevalence in older adults and is associated with significant adverse consequences. Several gaps in knowledge include the pathophysiology and consequences of SDB (**Box 1**). Alternate pathophysiology-based personalized therapies are required.

REFERENCES

1. The World Health Organization. World report on ageing and health. 2015. Available at: http://www.who.int/ageing/en/. Accessed January 30, 2017.
2. Carskadon MA, Dement WC. Respiration during sleep in the aged human. J Gerontol 1981;36(4):420–3.
3. Ancoli-Israel S, Kripke DF, Klauber MR, et al. Sleep-disordered breathing in community-dwelling elderly. Sleep 1991;14(6):486.
4. Hoch C, Reynolds C 3rd, Monk T, et al. Comparison of sleep-disordered breathing among healthy elderly in the seventh, eighth, and ninth decades of life. Sleep 1990;13(6):502–11.
5. Bixler EO, Vgontzas AN, Ten Have T, et al. Effects of age on sleep apnea in men: I. Prevalence and severity. Am J Respir Crit Care Med 1998;157(1):144–8.
6. Duran J, Esnaola S, Rubio R, et al. Obstructive sleep apnea-hypopnea and related clinical features in a population-based sample of subjects aged 30 to 70 yr. Am J Respir Crit Care Med 2001;163(3 Pt 1):685–9.
7. Bixler EO, Vgontzas AN, Lin H-M, et al. Prevalence of sleep-disordered breathing in women: effects of gender. Am J Respir Crit Care Med 2001;163(3):608–13.
8. Mehra R, Stone KL, Blackwell T, et al. Prevalence and correlates of sleep-disordered breathing in older men: osteoporotic fractures in men sleep study. J Am Geriatr Soc 2007;55(9):1356–64.
9. Young T, Palta M, Dempsey J, et al. The occurrence of sleep-disordered breathing among middle-aged adults. N Engl J Med 1993;328(17):1230–5.
10. Yeh NC, Tien KJ, Yang CM, et al. Increased risk of Parkinson's disease in patients with obstructive sleep apnea: a population-based, propensity score-matched, longitudinal follow-up study. Medicine (Baltimore) 2016;95(2):e2293.
11. Redline S, Schluchter MD, Larkin EK, et al. Predictors of longitudinal change in sleep-disordered breathing in a nonclinic population. Sleep 2003;26(6):703–9.
12. Young T, Finn L, Peppard PE, et al. Sleep disordered breathing and mortality: eighteen-year

follow-up of the Wisconsin sleep cohort. Sleep 2008;31(8):1071–8.

13. Fragoso CAV, Araujo KL, Van Ness PH, et al. Prevalence of sleep disturbances in a cohort of older drivers. J Gerontol A Biol Sci Med Sci 2008;63(7):715–23.

14. Kleisiaris CF, Kritsotakis EI, Daniil Z, et al. The prevalence of obstructive sleep apnea-hypopnea syndrome-related symptoms and their relation to airflow limitation in an elderly population receiving home care. Int J Chron Obstruct Pulmon Dis 2014;9:1111–7.

15. Onen F, Moreau T, Gooneratne NS, et al. Limits of the Epworth sleepiness scale in older adults. Sleep Breath 2013;17(1):343–50.

16. Nguyen-Michel VH, Lévy PP, Pallanca O, et al. Underperception of naps in older adults referred for a sleep assessment: an insomnia trait and a cognitive problem? J Am Geriatr Soc 2015;63(10):2001–7.

17. Fung CH, Martin JL, Dzierzewski JM, et al. Prevalence and symptoms of occult sleep disordered breathing among older veterans with insomnia. J Clin Sleep Med 2013;9(11):1173.

18. Young T, Shahar E, Nieto FJ, et al. Predictors of sleep-disordered breathing in community-dwelling adults: the sleep heart health study. Arch Intern Med 2002;162(8):893–900.

19. Degache F, Sforza E, Dauphinot V, et al. Relation of central fat mass to obstructive sleep apnea in the elderly. Sleep 2013;36(4):501–7.

20. Kleisiaris CF, Kritsotakis EI, Daniil Z, et al. Assessing the risk of obstructive sleep apnoea-hypopnoea syndrome in elderly home care patients with chronic multimorbidity: a cross-sectional screening study. Springerplus 2016;5:34.

21. Ancoli-Israel S, Kripke DF, Mason W, et al. Comparisons of home sleep recordings and polysomnograms in older adults with sleep disorders. Sleep 1981;4(3):283–91.

22. Morales CR, Hurley S, Wick LC, et al. In-home, self-assembled sleep studies are useful in diagnosing sleep apnea in the elderly. Sleep 2012;35(11):1491–501.

23. Pack AI, Silage DA, Millman RP, et al. Spectral analysis of ventilation in elderly subjects awake and asleep. J Appl Physiol (1985) 1988;64(3):1257–67.

24. Pack A, Cola M, Goldszmidt A, et al. Correlation between oscillations in ventilation and frequency content of the electroencephalogram. J Appl Physiol (1985) 1992;72(3):985–92.

25. Chowdhuri S, Pranathiageswaran S, Loomis-King H, et al. Aging is associated with Increased Propensity for Central Apnea during NREM Sleep. J Appl Physiol (1985) 2017. https://doi.org/10.1152/japplphysiol.00125.2017.

26. Wellman A, Malhotra A, Jordan AS, et al. Chemical control stability in the elderly. J Physiol 2007;581(Pt 1):291–8.

27. Poulin MJ, Cunningham D, Paterson D, et al. Ventilatory sensitivity to CO2 in hyperoxia and hypoxia in older aged humans. J Appl Physiol (1985) 1993;75(5):2209–16.

28. Chapman KR, Cherniack NS. Aging effects on the interaction of hypercapnia and hypoxia as ventilatory stimuli. J Gerontol 1987;42(2):202–9.

29. Browne H, Adams L, Simonds A, et al. Ageing does not influence the sleep-related decrease in the hypercapnic ventilatory response. Eur Respir J 2003;21(3):523–9.

30. Chowdhuri S, Pranathiageswaran S, Franco-Elizondo R, et al. Effect of age on long-term facilitation and chemosensitivity during NREM sleep. J Appl Physiol (1985) 2015;119(10):1088–96.

31. Lu H, Xu F, Rodrigue KM, et al. Alterations in cerebral metabolic rate and blood supply across the adult lifespan. Cereb Cortex 2011;21(6):1426–34.

32. Mayhan WG, Arrick DM, Sharpe GM, et al. Age-related alterations in reactivity of cerebral arterioles: role of oxidative stress. Microcirculation 2008;15(3):225–36.

33. Ballanyi K, Onimaru H, Homma I. Respiratory network function in the isolated brainstem-spinal cord of newborn rats. Prog Neurobiol 1999;59(6):583–634.

34. Martin S, Mathur R, Marshall I, et al. The effect of age, sex, obesity and posture on upper airway size. Eur Respir J 1997;10(9):2087–90.

35. Malhotra A, Huang Y, Fogel R, et al. Aging influences on pharyngeal anatomy and physiology: the predisposition to pharyngeal collapse. Am J Med 2006;119(1)(72):e79.

36. Eikermann M, Jordan AS, Chamberlin NL, et al. The influence of aging on pharyngeal collapsibility during sleep. Chest 2007;131(6):1702–9.

37. Burger CD, Stanson AW, Sheedy PF 2nd, et al. Fast-computed tomography evaluation of age-related changes in upper airway structure and function in normal men. Am Rev Respir Dis 1992;145(4 Pt 1):846–52.

38. Klawe JJ, Tafil-Klawe M. Age-related response of the genioglossus muscle EMG-activity to hypoxia in humans. J Physiol Pharmacol 2003;54(Suppl 1):14–9.

39. Edwards BA, Wellman A, Sands SA, et al. Obstructive sleep apnea in older adults is a distinctly different physiological phenotype. Sleep 2014;37(7):1227–36.

40. Strand LB, Carnethon M, Biggs ML, et al. Sleep disturbances and glucose metabolism in older adults: the cardiovascular health study. Diabetes Care 2015;38(11):2050–8.

41. Lavie L, Lavie P. Ischemic preconditioning as a possible explanation for the age decline relative

mortality in sleep apnea. Med Hypotheses 2006; 66(6):1069–73.

42. Haas DC, Foster GL, Nieto FJ, et al. Age-dependent associations between sleep-disordered breathing and hypertension importance of discriminating between systolic/diastolic hypertension and isolated systolic hypertension in the sleep heart health study. Circulation 2005;111(5):614–21.

43. Goff EA, O Driscoll DM, Simonds AK, et al. The cardiovascular response to arousal from sleep decreases with age in healthy adults. Sleep 2008; 31(7):1009.

44. Guillot M, Sforza E, Achour-Crawford E, et al. Association between severe obstructive sleep apnea and incident arterial hypertension in the older people population. Sleep Med 2013;14(9):838–42.

45. Fung MM, Peters K, Redline S, et al. Decreased slow wave sleep increases risk of developing hypertension in elderly men. Hypertension 2011; 58(4):596–603.

46. Nieto FJ, Young TB, Lind BK, et al. Association of sleep-disordered breathing, sleep apnea, and hypertension in a large community-based study. JAMA 2000;283(14):1829–36.

47. Yaggi HK, Concato J, Kernan WN, et al. Obstructive sleep apnea as a risk factor for stroke and death. N Engl J Med 2005;353(19):2034–41.

48. Punjabi NM, Caffo BS, Goodwin JL, et al. Sleep-disordered breathing and mortality: a prospective cohort study. PLoS Med 2009;6(8):e1000132.

49. Gottlieb DJ, Yenokyan G, Newman AB, et al. Prospective study of obstructive sleep apnea and incident coronary heart disease and heart failure: the sleep heart health study. Circulation 2010;122(4): 352–60.

50. Tuohy CV, Montez-Rath ME, Turakhia M, et al. Sleep disordered breathing and cardiovascular risk in older patients initiating dialysis in the United States: a retrospective observational study using Medicare data. BMC Nephrol 2016;17:16.

51. Javaheri S, Sharma RK, Wang R, et al. Association between obstructive sleep apnea and left ventricular structure by age and gender: the multi-ethnic study of atherosclerosis. Sleep 2016;39(3):523–9.

52. Ancoli-Israel S, DuHamel ER, Stepnowsky C, et al. The relationship between congestive heart failure, sleep apnea, and mortality in older men. Chest 2003;124(4):1400–5.

53. Martínez-García M-A, Campos-Rodríguez F, Catalán-Serra P, et al. Cardiovascular mortality in obstructive sleep apnea in the elderly: role of long-term continuous positive airway pressure treatment: a prospective observational study. Am J Respir Crit Care Med 2012;186(9):909–16.

54. Gooneratne NS, Richards KC, Joffe M, et al. Sleep disordered breathing with excessive daytime sleepiness is a risk factor for mortality in older adults. Sleep 2011;34(4):435–42.

55. Javaheri S, Blackwell T, Ancoli-Israel S, et al. Sleep-disordered breathing and incident heart failure in older men. Am J Respir Crit Care Med 2016; 193(5):561–8.

56. Mehra R, Stone KL, Varosy PD, et al. Nocturnal arrhythmias across a spectrum of obstructive and central sleep-disordered breathing in older men: outcomes of sleep disorders in older men (MrOS sleep) study. Arch Intern Med 2009;169(12): 1147–55.

57. May AM, Blackwell T, Stone PH, et al. Central sleep-disordered breathing predicts incident atrial fibrillation in older men. Am J Respir Crit Care Med 2016;193(7):783–91.

58. Stone KL, Blackwell TL, Ancoli-Israel S, et al. Sleep disordered breathing and risk of stroke in older community-dwelling men. Sleep 2015;39(3):531–40.

59. Munoz R, Duran-Cantolla J, Martínez-Vila E, et al. Severe sleep apnea and risk of ischemic stroke in the elderly. Stroke 2006;37(9):2317–21.

60. Yaffe K, Laffan AM, Harrison SL, et al. Sleep-disordered breathing, hypoxia, and risk of mild cognitive impairment and dementia in older women. JAMA 2011;306(6):613–9.

61. Zhou J, Camacho M, Tang X, et al. A review of neurocognitive function and obstructive sleep apnea with or without daytime sleepiness. Sleep Med 2016;23:99–108.

62. Alchanatis M, Zias N, Deligiorgis N, et al. Comparison of cognitive performance among different age groups in patients with obstructive sleep apnea. Sleep Breath 2008;12(1):17–24.

63. Aloia MS, Ilniczky N, Di Dio P, et al. Neuropsychological changes and treatment compliance in older adults with sleep apnea. J Psychosom Res 2003; 54(1):71–6.

64. Sforza E, Roche F, Thomas-Anterion C, et al. Cognitive function and sleep related breathing disorders in a healthy elderly population: the SYNAPSE study. Sleep 2010;33(4):515–21.

65. Blackwell T, Yaffe K, Laffan A, et al. Associations between sleep-disordered breathing, nocturnal hypoxemia, and subsequent cognitive decline in older community-dwelling men: the osteoporotic fractures in men sleep study. J Am Geriatr Soc 2015;63(3):453–61.

66. Martin MS, Sforza E, Roche F, et al, PROOF study group. Sleep breathing disorders and cognitive function in the elderly: an 8-year follow-up study. the proof-synapse cohort. Sleep 2015;38(2): 179–87.

67. Martin MS, Sforza E, Crawford-Achour E, et al. Sleep breathing disorders and cognitive decline in healthy elderly followed for eight years: the

PROOF cohort. Ann Phys Rehabil Med 2016;59S: e99.

68. Spira AP, Blackwell T, Stone KL, et al. Sleep-disordered breathing and cognition in older women. J Am Geriatr Soc 2008;56(1):45–50.

69. Ju G, Yoon IY, Lee SD, et al. Effects of sleep apnea syndrome on delayed memory and executive function in elderly adults. J Am Geriatr Soc 2012;60(6): 1099–103.

70. Hongyo K, Ito N, Yamamoto K, et al. Factors associated with the severity of obstructive sleep apnea in older adults. Geriatr Gerontol Int 2017;17(4): 614–21.

71. Rostanski SK, Zimmerman ME, Schupf N, et al. Sleep disordered breathing and white matter hyperintensities in community-dwelling elders. Sleep 2016;39(4):785–91.

72. Baril A-A, Gagnon K, Brayet P, et al. Gray matter hypertrophy and thickening with obstructive sleep apnea in middle-aged and older adults. Am J Respir Crit Care Med 2017;195(11):1509–18.

73. Daulatzai MA. Death by a thousand cuts in Alzheimer's disease: hypoxia–the prodrome. Neurotox Res 2013;24(2):216–43.

74. Alcántara C, Biggs ML, Davidson KW, et al. Sleep disturbances and depression in the multi-ethnic study of atherosclerosis. Sleep 2015; 39(4):915–25.

75. Farajzadeh M, Hosseini M, Mohtashami J, et al. The association between obstructive sleep apnea and depression in older adults. Nurs Midwifery Stud 2016;5(2):e32585.

76. Johansson P, Svensson E, Alehagen U, et al. Sleep disordered breathing, hypoxia and inflammation: associations with sickness behaviour in community dwelling elderly with and without cardiovascular disease. Sleep Breath 2015;19(1):263–71.

77. Sforza E, de Saint Hilaire Z, Pelissolo A, et al. Personality, anxiety and mood traits in patients with sleep-related breathing disorders: effect of reduced daytime alertness. Sleep Med 2002;3(2): 139–45.

78. Sforza E, Saint Martin M, Barthélémy JC, et al. Mood disorders in healthy elderly with obstructive sleep apnea: a gender effect. Sleep Med 2016; 19:57–62.

79. Moon K, Punjabi NM, Aurora RN. Obstructive sleep apnea and type 2 diabetes in older adults. Clin Geriatr Med 2015;31(1):139–47.

80. Spira AP, Stone KL, Rebok GW, et al. Sleep-disordered breathing and functional decline in older women. J Am Geriatr Soc 2014;62(11):2040–6.

81. Sandberg M, Kristensson J, Midlov P, et al. Prevalence and predictors of healthcare utilization among older people (60+): focusing on ADL dependency and risk of depression. Arch Gerontol Geriatr 2012;54(3):e349–63.

82. Tarasiuk A, Greenberg-Dotan S, Simon-Tuval T, et al. The effect of obstructive sleep apnea on morbidity and health care utilization of middle-aged and older adults. J Am Geriatr Soc 2008; 56(2):247–54.

83. Stepnowsky C, Johnson S, Dimsdale J, et al. Sleep apnea and health-related quality of life in African-American elderly. Ann Behav Med 2000;22(2): 116–20.

84. Martínez-García M, Soler-Cataluna J, Román-Sánchez P, et al. Obstructive sleep apnea has little impact on quality of life in the elderly. Sleep Med 2009;10(1):104–11.

85. Kostikas K, Browne HA, Ghiassi R, et al. The determinants of therapeutic levels of continuous positive airway pressure in elderly sleep apnea patients. Respir Med 2006;100(7):1216–25.

86. Ayalon L, Ancoli-Israel S, Stepnowsky C, et al. Adherence to continuous positive airway pressure treatment in patients with Alzheimer disease and obstructive sleep apnea. Am J Geriatr Psychiatry 2006;14(2):176–80.

87. Chong MS, Ayalon L, Marler M, et al. Continuous positive airway pressure reduces subjective daytime sleepiness in patients with mild to moderate Alzheimer's disease with sleep disordered breathing. J Am Geriatr Soc 2006;54(5):777–81.

88. Pelletier-Fleury N, Rakotonanahary D, Fleury B. The age and other factors in the evaluation of compliance with nasal continuous positive airway pressure for obstructive sleep apnea syndrome. A Cox's proportional hazard analysis. Sleep Med 2001;2(3):225–32.

89. Russo-Magno P, O'Brien A, Panciera T, et al. Compliance with CPAP therapy in older men with obstructive sleep apnea. J Am Geriatr Soc 2001; 49(9):1205–11.

90. Aloia MS, Di Dio L, Ilniczky N, et al. Improving compliance with nasal CPAP and vigilance in older adults with OSAHS. Sleep Breath 2001;5(1):13–22.

91. Marin JM, Carrizo SJ, Vicente E, et al. Long-term cardiovascular outcomes in men with obstructive sleep apnoea-hypopnoea with or without treatment with continuous positive airway pressure: an observational study. Lancet 2005;365(9464): 1046–53.

92. Campos-Rodriguez F, Martinez-Garcia MA, de la Cruz-Moron I, et al. Cardiovascular mortality in women with obstructive sleep apnea with or without continuous positive airway pressure treatment: a cohort study. Ann Intern Med 2012; 156(2):115–22.

93. López-Padilla D, Alonso-Moralejo R, Martínez-García MÁ, et al. Continuous positive airway pressure and survival of very elderly persons with moderate to severe obstructive sleep apnea. Sleep Med 2016;19:23–9.

94. McMillan A, Bratton DJ, Faria R, et al. Continuous positive airway pressure in older people with obstructive sleep apnoea syndrome (PREDICT): a 12-month, multicentre, randomised trial. Lancet Respir Med 2014;2(10):804–12.

95. Carballo NJ, Alessi CA, Martin JL, et al. Perceived effectiveness, self-efficacy, and social support for oral appliance therapy among older veterans with obstructive sleep apnea. Clin Ther 2016;38(11): 2407–15.

96. Endeshaw YW, White WB, Kutner M, et al. Sleep-disordered breathing and 24-hour blood pressure pattern among older adults. J Gerontol A Biol Sci Med Sci 2009;64(2):280–5.

97. Mant A, King M, Saunders NA, et al. Four-year follow-up of mortality and sleep-related respiratory disturbance in non-demented seniors. Sleep 1995; 18(6):433–8.

98. Martinez-Garcia MA, Soler-Cataluna JJ, Ejarque-Martinez L, et al. Continuous positive airway pressure treatment reduces mortality in patients with ischemic stroke and obstructive sleep apnea: a 5-year follow-up study. Am J Respir Crit Care Med 2009;180(1):36–41.

99. Johansson P, Alehagen U, Svanborg E, et al. Clinical characteristics and mortality risk in relation to obstructive and central sleep apnoea in community-dwelling elderly individuals: a 7-year follow-up. Age Ageing 2012;41(4):468–74.

100. Holmqvist F, Guan N, Zhu Z, et al. Impact of obstructive sleep apnea and continuous positive airway pressure therapy on outcomes in patients with atrial fibrillation-results from the Outcomes Registry for Better Informed Treatment of Atrial Fibrillation (ORBIT-AF). Am Heart J 2015;169(5):647–54.e642.

101. Lim AS, Kowgier M, Yu L, et al. Sleep fragmentation and the risk of incident Alzheimer's disease and cognitive decline in older persons. Sleep 2013; 36(7):1027–32.

Circadian Rhythm Sleep-Wake Disorders in Older Adults

 CrossMark

Jee Hyun Kim, MD, PhD[a,b,c], Jeanne F. Duffy, MBA, PhD[b,c],*

KEYWORDS

- Circadian rhythm sleep disorders • Advanced sleep phase • Delayed sleep phase • Melatonin
- Circadian rhythm disruption • Alzheimer disease • Light therapy

KEY POINTS

- The circadian timing system regulates the timing, structure, and consolidation of sleep, in conjunction with a sleep-wake homeostatic process.
- There are age-related changes in the circadian regulation of sleep, in the sleep homeostatic regulation of sleep, and in the interaction between these two processes.
- Circadian rhythm sleep-wake disorders result from a mismatch between the desired timing of sleep and the ability to fall asleep or remain asleep.
- Advanced sleep-wake phase disorder and irregular sleep-wake rhythm disorder are more common in older adults than in young adults.
- Jet lag disorder and shift-work disorder are more commonly experienced by travelers and workers as they age.

INTRODUCTION

The timing, duration, and consolidation of human sleep result largely from the interaction of 2 sleep regulatory systems: the sleep-wake homeostat and the circadian timing system. When these 2 processes are aligned and functioning optimally, they allow adults to achieve a long, consolidated bout of wakefulness throughout the day and a long and consolidated sleep episode at night. Changes to either process, or a change in how the 2 processes interact, can result in an inability to fall asleep at the desired time, difficulty remaining asleep, or difficulty remaining awake throughout the desired wake episode. This mismatch between the desired timing of sleep (and wakefulness) and the ability to fall asleep and remain asleep is a hallmark of a distinct class of sleep disorders called the circadian rhythm sleep-wake disorders (CRSWDs). This article discusses the circadian timing system, the role played by the circadian system in sleep-wake regulation, typical changes in circadian regulation of sleep with aging, the CRSWDs and how age influences their diagnosis and treatment, and how neurologic diseases in older patients affect circadian rhythms and sleep.

Disclosure: J.H. Kim was supported by a grant from Dankook University; J.F. Duffy supported by NIH grants R01 AG044416 and P01 AG09975.
[a] Department of Neurology, Dankook University College of Medicine, Dankook University Hospital, Manghyang-ro 201, Dongnam-gu, Cheonan, Chungnam 31116, Republic of Korea; [b] Division of Sleep and Circadian Disorders, Departments of Medicine and Neurology, Brigham and Women's Hospital, 221 Longwood Avenue, BLI438, Boston, MA 02115, USA; [c] Division of Sleep Medicine, Harvard Medical School, Boston, MA, USA
* Corresponding author. Division of Sleep and Circadian Disorders, Brigham and Women's Hospital, 221 Longwood Avenue BLI438, Boston, MA 02115.
E-mail address: jduffy@research.bwh.harvard.edu

Sleep Med Clin 13 (2018) 39–50
https://doi.org/10.1016/j.jsmc.2017.09.004

CIRCADIAN RHYTHM SLEEP-WAKE DISORDERS

Although surveys[1] suggest that less than 3% of the adult population have a CRSWD, the CRSWDs are often confused with insomnia, resulting in underestimates of the true prevalence. Some estimates are that up to 10% of adult patients with sleep disorders may have a CRSWD.[2] Although some CRSWDs (such as jet lag) can be self-limiting, others, when untreated, can lead to adverse medical, psychological, and social consequences for affected patients. The International Classification of Sleep Disorders classifies CRSWDs as disorders related to the timing of sleep and wakefulness, with 6 subtypes[3]: delayed sleep-wake phase disorder, advanced sleep-wake phase disorder, irregular sleep-wake rhythm disorder, non-24-hour sleep-wake rhythm disorder, jet lag disorder, and shift-work disorder (**Table 1**). The primary clinical characteristic of all CRSWDs is an inability to fall asleep, remain asleep, and/or wake at the desired time. CRSWDs arise from a problem with the internal biological clock (circadian timing system) and/or misalignment between the circadian timing system and the external 24-hour environment. This misalignment can be the result of biological and/or behavioral factors, and the rates of different CRSWDs vary across age groups.

THE CIRCADIAN TIMING SYSTEM IN HUMANS

The circadian timing system refers to near–24-hour rhythmicity in many aspects of physiology and behavior, including not only sleep and waking but hormone secretion, body temperature, and urine production.[4–6] These rhythms are features of individual cells[7] and arise through transcription-translation feedback loops.[8] Coordination of the rhythms among cells within an organ, and between the organ systems of the body, are achieved through signals from a master pacemaker in the hypothalamus, the suprachiasmatic nucleus (SCN).[9] The SCN not only coordinates the rhythmic activity of the cells and organs within the body but synchronizes the near–24-hour rhythmic activity of the body with the 24-hour cycle of the external environment, a process called entrainment. A functional circadian timing system allows the organism to predict regular changes that occur in the environment (eg, sunlight, food availability, presence of predators) and to prepare for those changes, thus providing an adaptive advantage.[10]

Because the underlying rhythmicity is close to, but not exactly, 24 hours in cycle length, it must be synchronized or entrained to the external 24-hour day on a regular basis. Entrainment of the near–24-hour circadian system to the 24-hour day occurs typically through exposure to signals from the environment, and in the case of humans (as in most other mammals) this is largely done via regular exposure to light during the day and darkness at night. Studies in healthy sighted adults have shown that the period (cycle length) of the circadian system averages around 24.2 hours across age groups.[11] This finding implies that the average adult's circadian system needs to be reset about 10 minutes earlier each day in order to remain synchronized to external clock time, and, if it is not, then the circadian system may drift out of synchrony with external clock time. One example of this desynchronization is what happens to many blind individuals. They complain of cyclic sleep-wake problems, alternating periods when they can sleep well at night and are alert during the day with times when their nighttime sleep is disturbed and they struggle to remain awake throughout the day.[12]

Although on average the circadian period is 24.2 hours, the range between individuals is about an hour, from approximately 23.5 to 24.5 hours,[11] which means that individuals with the shortest and longest periods need to reset by half an hour each day to remain entrained, and, without that regular resetting, they are even more likely than the average person to drift out of synchronization. Individuals with the shortest and longest periods are therefore most susceptible to non-24-hour sleep-wake rhythm disorder. On average, the circadian period in women is shorter than in men, and significantly more women than men have a period that is less than 24 hours.[11] This difference predisposes women to advanced sleep-wake phase disorder.

CIRCADIAN REGULATION OF SLEEP AND WAKEFULNESS

Key points
- The circadian timing system coregulates the timing, structure, and consolidation of sleep
- The circadian timing system interacts with the sleep-wake homeostat to allow consolidated wakefulness during the day and consolidated sleep at night

The circadian system is a major determinant of the timing of sleep and internal sleep structure in humans.[13] Specialized experimental techniques have been used to separate the circadian and sleep-wake homeostatic influences on sleep in order to understand how each independently influences sleep and wakefulness. Those studies have revealed that although most aspects of sleep are influenced by the biological time at which sleep

Table 1
Characteristics of individual circadian rhythm sleep-wake disorders with special considerations for older patients

Circadian Rhythm Sleep-Wake Disorder	Basic Characteristics	Age-Related Considerations
Delayed sleep-wake phase disorder	Sleep timing that occurs later than desired or required	Less common in older adults
Advanced sleep-wake phase disorder	Sleep timing that occurs earlier than desired or required	More common in older adults
Irregular sleep-wake rhythm disorder	Irregularity in sleep-wake timing, often including multiple irregular short sleep bouts within a day	More common in older adults, particularly in the context of dementia
Non–24-h sleep-wake rhythm disorder	Sleep timing that moves progressively later each night (or, rarely, moves earlier each night)	More common in older adults, particularly in the context of vision loss
Jet lag disorder	An inability to sleep at night and/or remain awake throughout the day after traveling across several time zones. This condition is caused by the abrupt mismatch between internal biological time and external time resulting from rapid travel across time zones, and is typically self-limiting	Older adults more affected because of decreased ability to sleep at adverse circadian time
Shift-work disorder	Characterized by an inability to obtain sufficient sleep during the day and difficulty remaining awake at night resulting from night work. Shift-work disorder can also affect day workers whose early morning shifts require very early rise times	Older adults may be more susceptible to the negative impacts of shift work on sleep

All CRSWDs are characterized by an inability to fall asleep, remain asleep, and/or awaken at the desired or required times.

occurs, the circadian system has its strongest impact on rapid eye movement (REM) sleep, sleep latency, and sleep consolidation.[14] The rhythm in circadian sleep-wake propensity is such that the strongest drive for wakefulness occurs in the evening, close to the end of the usual wake episode (creating the wake maintenance zone or forbidden zone for sleep). Similarly, the strongest drive for sleep occurs in the late night/early morning hours, close to the time of the end of the usual sleep episode. When this rhythm in sleep-wake propensity interacts with the sleep-wake homeostatic process, it results in an ability to remain awake across a long episode each day, and to remain asleep for a long and consolidated time each night. Laboratory studies have shown that the ability to have a long consolidated sleep episode is critically dependent on the proper alignment of the timing of sleep with respect to the underlying circadian rhythm of sleep-wake propensity.[14,15] Misalignment, such as occurs when night-shift workers attempt to

sleep during the day, typically produces an inability to sleep for more than a few hours,[16] and can result in shift-work disorder.

AGE-RELATED CHANGES IN CIRCADIAN RHYTHMS

Key points
- There are age-related changes in the phase (timing) of circadian rhythms
- There are age-related changes in the amplitude of circadian rhythms
- There are age-related changes how the circadian and sleep homeostatic systems interact
- With advancing age, the ability to sleep at adverse circadian phases is compromised, even in healthy individuals

The timing of the circadian rhythms of body temperature, melatonin, and cortisol have been shown to move earlier, or advance, in older adults compared with young adults.[17] In addition, there are numerous reports that the amplitude of circadian rhythms, including those of body temperature, melatonin, and other hormones, are reduced in older adults.[17] Studies in animals suggest that these age-related changes in rhythms may be caused by changes in the SCN.[18] In addition to changes in the timing of physiologic rhythms controlled by the circadian timing system, there are also reports that the relative timing of rhythms with respect to sleep-wake timing change with age.[19] This latter finding means that older adults are not only sleeping at different clock times than young adults, they are also sleeping at different biological times.

Laboratory studies have shown that the sleep of older adults is much more sensitive to the circadian time at which it occurs than is the sleep of young adults,[15] thus making older adults more vulnerable to the CRSWDs jet lag disorder and shift-work disorder (discussed later). Studies in which the circadian time of sleep is systematically manipulated have revealed that there may be an age-related reduction in the amplitude of the circadian rhythm of sleep-wake propensity that not only makes it more difficult to sleep at an adverse circadian time but makes consolidation of an extended nighttime sleep episode more difficult.[15,20]

DIAGNOSIS OF CIRCADIAN RHYTHM SLEEP-WAKE DISORDERS

As described earlier, CRSWDs are assumed to result from a mismatch between the timing of sleep (and wakefulness) and the underlying circadian rhythm of sleep-wake propensity. Despite this, current standards[3,21] for diagnosis of a CRSWD do not require assessment of circadian rhythmicity but instead focus on the timing of sleep alone. This lack of circadian rhythm assessment may contribute to the poor treatment outcomes of some patients with CRSWDs.[22]

Diagnosis of all CRSWDs requires that 3 main criteria are met:

- The complaint is chronic
- The affected patient has problems with sleep (difficulty falling asleep, difficulty remaining asleep, or waking too early), difficulty remaining awake (excessive daytime sleepiness), or both
- The sleep-wake problem causes clinically significant distress or impairment of 1 or more areas of functioning

Depending on the CRSWD, there are additional and/or specific criteria used to make a diagnosis. These are outlined in **Box 1**.

PREVALENCE OF CIRCADIAN RHYTHM SLEEP-WAKE DISORDERS IN OLDER ADULTS

Key points

- Although CRSWD diagnoses are not common, older adults are much more likely than young adults to be diagnosed with advanced sleep-wake phase disorder and irregular sleep-wake rhythm disorder
- Older individuals are more prone to jet lag disorder and shift-work disorder than their younger counterparts (and even more prone than when they were younger) because of a reduced ability to sleep at adverse circadian phases

Early morning awakening (EMA) is common among older adults.[23] Although some surveys of older adults indicate that 20% to 30% of them report EMA, when individuals with comorbidities such as depression, pain, physical limitations, and respiratory symptoms are excluded, less than 4% of those remaining have EMA.[24] It is impossible to determine from these subjective complaints whether circadian changes underlie the EMA, although in some cases the EMA meets the criteria for advanced sleep-wake phase disorder.

Advanced sleep-wake phase disorder, although rare, is found more frequently in older adults than in young adults.[1,25] As outlined in **Box 1**, delayed sleep-wake phase disorder is found rarely in older adults.[25,26] Non–24-hour sleep-wake rhythm disorder, although rare in sighted older adults, may develop secondary to loss of vision.[27] Irregular sleep-wake rhythm disorder is also rare and is found most frequently in patients with dementias and in institutionalized individuals,[28] likely in part because of the lack of strong daily environmental and behavioral influences that typically synchronize circadian rhythms.[29] Jet lag disorder and shift-work disorder may affect individuals to a greater extent as they age,[30,31] because of typical age-related changes in sleep. This greater effect is because the sleep of older adults, even those who are in good health and without sleep disorders, is more vulnerable to misalignment with the circadian rhythm of sleep-wake propensity.[15,19,20] As a consequence, older shift workers report more sleep problems and have higher rates of hypnotic use than younger shift workers.[32]

NEUROLOGIC IMPLICATIONS OF CIRCADIAN RHYTHM CHANGES IN OLDER ADULTS

Key points

- Patients with neurodegenerative diseases show changes in rest-activity patterns and sleep disruptions, and these may be caused by circadian disruption

Box 1
Diagnostic criteria for circadian rhythm sleep-wake disorders that are most common in older adults

Main criteria for all CRSWDs:

- The sleep-wake complaint is chronic
- The patient has a problem with sleep (difficulty falling asleep, remaining asleep, or waking too early), difficulty remaining awake (excessive daytime sleepiness), or both
- The sleep-wake problem causes clinically significant distress or impairment of 1 or more areas of daytime functioning

Advanced sleep-wake phase disorder, additional criteria:

- An advance in the timing of sleep relative to the desired or required timing, both by history and as shown using actigraphy and/or a daily sleep log for at least 1 week
- Symptoms/complaint present for at least 3 months
- When allowed to sleep without timing constraints, the patient is able to achieve a sleep episode of good quality and sufficient duration, although the timing is advanced
- The sleep problem is not explained by any other sleep, medical, neurologic, or psychological disorder, by medication, or by substance use/abuse

Irregular sleep-wake rhythm disorder, additional criteria:

- Irregular sleep and wake episodes throughout the 24-hour day, both by history and as shown using actigraphy and/or a daily sleep log for at least 1 week; 3 or more sleep episodes per 24 hours; difficulty sleeping/remaining asleep at night; difficulty remaining awake during the day
- Symptoms/complaint present for at least 3 months
- The sleep problem is not explained by any other sleep, medical, neurologic, or psychological disorder, by medication, or by substance use/abuse

Shift-work disorder, additional criteria:

- When working a particular shift (night shift or day shift with early morning start time), difficulty sleeping and/or excessive sleepiness, with overall reduced sleep duration by history and as shown using actigraphy and/or a daily sleep log for at least 1 week
- Symptoms/complaint present for at least 3 months when on the work schedule
- The sleep problem is not explained by any other sleep, medical, neurologic, or psychological disorder, by medication, by substance use/abuse, or by the patient forgoing daytime sleep to work a second job or perform childcare or other activities

Jet lag disorder, additional criteria:

- Difficulty sleeping and/or excessive sleepiness, with overall reduced sleep duration following rapid travel across 2 or more time zones
- Impairment of function that develops within a few days of the travel
- The sleep problem is not explained by any other sleep, medical, neurologic, or psychological disorder, by medication, or by substance use/abuse

Note that assessment of endogenous circadian rhythmicity (eg, timing of evening melatonin secretion onset) is not required for diagnosis.
Data from American Academy of Sleep Medicine. International classification of sleep disorders. 3rd edition. Darien (IL): American Academy of Sleep Medicine; 2014.

- Changes in sleep may be an early sign of future neurodegenerative changes
- Changes in sleep often precede cognitive decline, and more severe sleep changes are associated with faster/greater cognitive decline
- Postoperative delirium, with associated sleep pattern changes, may be a warning sign for later cognitive decline

As described earlier, it is typical for older adults to experience circadian rhythm changes, and most often these changes go unrecognized unless they are accompanied by significant sleep disturbances or daytime dysfunction. However, there is growing evidence from numerous epidemiologic studies that sleep problems in older adults, including modest circadian rhythm changes, might represent an early sign of cognitive decline, potential development of a neurodegenerative disease, and might also be associated with increased mortality.[33–39] A bidirectional relationship between sleep and neurodegeneration has been suggested based on evidence from studies in animals.[40,41] These findings may relate to the recent discovery of the brain glymphatic system, hypothesized to be responsible for eliminating metabolic waste, including amyloid-β proteins, from the brain during sleep.[42]

How circadian rhythm changes are associated with the sleep-cognitive decline relationship are not well understood, because few studies have attempted to measure circadian rhythms.[34,36,37] Although actigraphy cannot assess the function of the underlying endogenous circadian pacemaker, rest-activity monitoring by actigraphy is the most commonly reported measure used to monitor the sleep-wake rhythm in older adults. Many studies have extracted variables from activity that are associated with cognitive changes, including interdaily stability (a measure of rest-activity rhythm synchronization to 24-hour clock time), intradaily variability (a measure of rhythm fragmentation), amplitude, as well as acrophase or nadir of activity.[36,37,43–45] Whether those rest-activity changes relate to changes in the circadian timing system remains to be determined. However, 2 studies of patients with probable Alzheimer disease (AD) found that the acrophase (ie, timing of the rhythm peak) of the core body temperature rhythms of patients with AD was delayed compared with controls,[46,47] suggesting that there may be circadian changes that underlie the sleep-wake changes.

Another hint that changes in sleep-wake behavior are associated with subsequent cognitive decline occurs in patients experiencing delirium during hospitalization or after major surgery. The sleep-wake behavior in patients experiencing delirium shares similar features with sundown syndrome/day-night reversal. One study followed the cognitive status in previously high-functioning patients who experienced postoperative delirium during a hospital stay and found that they showed an approximately 3-fold greater rate of decline of cognition in the 36 months after surgery.[48] Difficulty falling asleep in community-dwelling older adults is also associated with memory problems,[24] and thus these 2 lines of evidence hint that a phase delay or circadian disruption, manifested through altered sleep timing, is associated with cognitive decline. Whether the altered sleep timing (and presumed circadian alteration) is a cause or a symptom of the cognitive decline remains to be determined.

In summary, although it is not always clear that a change in rest-activity patterns represents a change in circadian rhythms, a delay of the rest-activity pattern seems to precede later cognitive decline in the older population. For otherwise healthy older patients who present features of a circadian rhythm sleep-wake disorder, especially a phase delay, careful assessment and monitoring of their cognitive statuses may be warranted, because the sleep-wake timing change may be an early indicator of neurodegenerative changes. Longitudinal studies with careful clinical observations that include robust sleep and circadian rhythm measures (such as melatonin secretion) will provide greater insights into how circadian and sleep changes may be associated with neurodegeneration.

CIRCADIAN RHYTHM DISRUPTION IN OLDER PATIENTS WITH NEURODEGENERATIVE DISEASE

Patients with neurodegenerative disease commonly present with sleep-wake disturbances and/or sleep disorders (including insomnia, excessive daytime sleepiness, sudden sleep attacks, and REM behavior disorder) at an early stage. These disorders may result from structural changes in the SCN and/or in the way SCN cells communicate,[18] because the SCN in patients with AD shows more severe changes compared with age-matched adults without AD.[49,50]

As described earlier, studies that have assessed the rhythm of core body temperature have found a significant delay of the rhythm in patients with probable[47] or actual AD.[51] Some studies have reported that disruption of rhythms in AD may be caused by pathologic changes to structures in the light input pathway from the eye to the SCN.[52–54]

Sleep disturbance is the most common nonmotor manifestation of Parkinson disease (PD), with an incidence of 60% to 80%.[55] Insomnia, dream-enacting behaviors, excessive daytime sleepiness, snoring/apnea, restless legs syndrome, and sudden sleep attacks are common sleep complaints. REM behavior disorder is now recognized as an important early nonmotor phenomenon associated with later development of PD and Parkinson-Plus syndrome. However, few studies have been done to evaluate circadian markers in patients with PD. Changes in phase and amplitude of the melatonin rhythm in patients with PD have been reported,[56,57] suggesting that circadian dysfunction may be a feature of PD. There are also reports of circadian alterations in other neurodegenerative disorders, such as progressive supranuclear palsy[58] and Huntington disease.[59–61]

In summary, patients with certain neurodegenerative diseases show sleep-wake changes, and there is some evidence that there may also be circadian changes. However, additional studies measuring circadian markers in connection with clinical features are needed to understand what role the circadian system plays in the sleep-wake changes associated with those neurodegenerative diseases.

TREATMENT OF CIRCADIAN SLEEP-WAKE DISORDERS IN OLDER ADULTS

Key points
- Treatments focus on resetting and/or synchronizing circadian rhythms
- Light therapy and/or melatonin are common strategies
- Much more research is needed to develop clinical guidelines and protocols for the use of light therapy and other treatments for CRSWDs in older adults

As outlined in **Table 2**, the most common treatments used for CRSWDs are designed to reset or synchronize the circadian timing system. A basic strategy used in all CRSWDs is to have the patients select a sleep time and attempt to strictly adhere to it. In addition, therapies that shift rhythm timing are often used, including bright light therapy and melatonin administration. In some cases, hypnotics to promote sleep and/or stimulants to promote wakefulness are also used.

LIGHT THERAPY

The timing of light exposure is crucial when using light therapy for the treatment of CRSWDs.[62–66] According to the phase response curves to light, evening/early night light delays circadian phase, whereas late night/early morning light advances circadian phase.[67] In young adults, duration-dependent responses to light have been reported,[68,69] with the maximal responses occurring in the initial minutes of light exposure. Najjar and Zeitzer[70] reported that intermittent flashes of light can produce significant circadian effects. Although additional studies in clinical populations need to be performed, such findings suggest that patients might not need to remain fixed in front of a light box to achieve phase shifts, improving practicality and compliance. In terms of the optimal intensity for light therapy, there are some reports that older adults may be less sensitive to light than young adults,[63,71,72] although not all studies have identified an age difference.[63,65]

There is evidence that light transmission is affected by typical age-related changes in the lens of the eye, which may contribute to differential impacts of light therapy between young and older adults.[73]

Despite findings from laboratory studies, there are few randomized trials in clinical populations that show the benefit of light therapy for older adults with advanced sleep-wake phase disorder,[74] and some studies show little to no impact.[75,76] Clinical treatment guidelines suggest that there is only weak evidence for evening light therapy in advanced sleep-wake phase disorder,[77] and there are no detailed guidelines for the intensity, duration, or timing for light therapy.

TREATMENT OF IRREGULAR SLEEP-WAKE RHYTHM DISORDER IN OLDER ADULTS

Irregular sleep-wake rhythm disorder in older adults is most common in patients with neurodegenerative disease, including AD and other dementias, especially as the disease advances. The disruptive impact of the irregular sleep pattern is one of the main reasons for institutionalization.[78,79] Several studies have been performed to test whether light interventions improve the fragmented sleep-wake patterns in such patients, with mixed results.[76,80–82] Combined light and melatonin interventions have also been tested, with some finding improvements in sleep and/or behavior.[83–85] Related interventions that include limits on daytime time in bed, increased light exposure during the day, and decreased disruptions at night (eg, noise, caregiver interventions) have been reported to improve sleep-wake function.[86]

TREATMENT OF SHIFT-WORK SLEEP DISORDER IN OLDER ADULTS

Older adults are reported to be less tolerant to shift work,[31,87] and this is typically attributed to the decreased ability of older individuals to sleep at an adverse circadian phase.[15]

Nonpharmacologic interventions to treat shift-work disorder include bright light exposure in the nighttime work environment and avoiding light on the morning commute home, strategic napping, as well as use of caffeine and other stimulants.[88–90] Although few of those studies have focused on older shift workers exclusively, a recent study found that a combined intervention of enhanced lighting and scheduled evening sleep was effective in improving night-shift alertness and performance in older individuals.[91] Additional studies testing interventions in older shift workers are needed.[92]

Table 2
Common treatments for circadian rhythm sleep-wake disorders

CRSWD	Common Recommendations and Treatments
Advanced sleep-wake phase disorder	• Adhere to a fixed sleep schedule • Evening bright light
Irregular sleep-wake rhythm disorder	• Adhere to a fixed sleep schedule • Daytime bright light • Evening melatonin
Non-24-h sleep-wake rhythm disorder	• Adhere to a fixed sleep schedule • Chronotherapy • Evening melatonin • Morning bright light exposure
Jet lag disorder	• Adhere to a fixed sleep schedule • Appropriately timed melatonin • Hypnotics • Timed light exposure (including minimizing exposure to bright light at certain times) • Caffeine and other stimulants
Shift-work disorder	• Timed light exposure (including minimizing exposure to bright light on the commute home in the morning) • Appropriately timed melatonin • Modafinil • Strategic napping • Caffeine

Data from Auger RR, Burgess HJ, Emens JS, et al. Clinical practice guideline for the treatment of intrinsic circadian rhythm sleep-wake disorders: advanced sleep-wake phase disorder (ASWPD), delayed sleep-wake phase disorder (DSWPD), non-24-hour sleep-wake rhythm disorder (N24SWD), and irregular sleep-wake rhythm disorder (ISWRD). An update for 2015: an American Academy of Sleep Medicine Clinical Practice Guideline. J Clin Sleep Med 2015;11(10):1199–236.

SUMMARY

The circadian timing system has a strong impact on the timing, structure, and consolidation of sleep, and interacts with a sleep-wake homeostatic process to allow extended sleep and wake episodes. With age, there are changes to both of these sleep regulatory processes, as well as a change in the way they interact. Those age-related changes in sleep make it more likely that older adults will experience certain CRSWDs, particularly advanced sleep-wake phase disorder, jet lag disorder, and shift-work disorder. In addition, other medical changes that occur with aging can contribute to a greater likelihood of the CRSWD irregular sleep-wake rhythm disorder. Although sleep hygiene, bright light therapy, melatonin administration, and other therapies are used to treat the CRSWDs, few systematic studies have been performed to determine the optimal strategy for treating CRSWDs, and few such studies have specifically tested the therapies in older adults. These deficiencies are compounded by current standards not requiring assessment of circadian rhythmicity in diagnosis of CRSWDs, mainly because of the time and expense of doing so.

Thus, there remain significant knowledge gaps in the diagnosis and treatment of CRSWDs, especially in older patients.[93]

ACKNOWLEDGMENTS

The authors thank Ms D. Mohan for assistance with the references.

REFERENCES

1. Schrader H, Bovim G, Sand T. The prevalence of delayed and advanced sleep phase syndromes. J Sleep Res 1993;2:51–5.
2. Barion A, Zee PC. A clinical approach to circadian rhythm sleep disorders. Sleep Med 2007;8(6): 566–77.
3. American Academy of Sleep Medicine. International classification of sleep disorders. 3rd edition. Darien (IL): American Academy of Sleep Medicine; 2014.
4. Czeisler CA, Klerman EB. Circadian and sleep-dependent regulation of hormone release in humans. Recent Prog Horm Res 1999;54:97–132.
5. Czeisler CA, Gooley JJ. Sleep and circadian rhythms in humans. Cold Spring Harb Symp Quant Biol 2007;72:579–97.

6. Czeisler CA, Buxton OM. Human circadian timing system and sleep-wake regulation. In: Kryger MH, Roth T, Dement WC, editors. Principles and practice of sleep medicine. 6th edition. Philadelphia: WB Saunders; 2017. p. 362–76.

7. Ko CH, Takahashi JS. Molecular components of the mammalian circadian clock. Hum Mol Genet 2006; 15(Spec No 2):R271–7.

8. Dibner C, Schibler U, Albrecht U. The mammalian circadian timing system: organization and coordination of central and peripheral clocks. Annu Rev Physiol 2010;72:517–49.

9. Menaker M, Takahashi JS, Eskin A. The physiology of circadian pacemakers. Annu Rev Physiol 1978; 40:501–26.

10. DeCoursey PJ. Survival value of suprachiasmatic nuclei (SCN) in four wild sciurid rodents. Behav Neurosci 2014;128(3):240–9.

11. Duffy JF, Cain SW, Chang AM, et al. Sex difference in the near-24-hour intrinsic period of the human circadian timing system. Proc Natl Acad Sci U S A 2011; 108(suppl. 3):15602–8.

12. Lockley SW, Arendt J, Skene DJ. Visual impairment and circadian rhythm disorders. Dialogues Clin Neurosci 2007;9(3):301–14.

13. Czeisler CA, Dijk DJ. Human circadian physiology and sleep-wake regulation. In: Takahashi JS, Turek FW, Moore RY, editors. Handbook of behavioral neurobiology: circadian clocks. New York: Plenum Publishing; 2001. p. 531–69.

14. Dijk DJ, Czeisler CA. Contribution of the circadian pacemaker and the sleep homeostat to sleep propensity, sleep structure, electroencephalographic slow waves, and sleep spindle activity in humans. J Neurosci 1995;15(5):3526–38.

15. Dijk DJ, Duffy JF, Riel E, et al. Ageing and the circadian and homeostatic regulation of human sleep during forced desynchrony of rest, melatonin and temperature rhythms. J Physiol 1999;516(2): 611–27.

16. Centers for Disease Control and Prevention (CDC). Short sleep duration among workers – United States, 2010. MMWR Morb Mortal Wkly Rep 2012;61(16): 281–5.

17. Duffy JF, Zitting KM, Chinoy ED. Aging and circadian rhythms. Sleep Med Clin 2015;10(4):423–34.

18. Engelberth RCGJ, Bezerra de Pontes AL, Porto Fiuza F, et al. Changes in the suprachiasmatic nucleus during aging: implications for biological rhythms. Psychology & Neuroscience 2013;6(3): 287–97.

19. Duffy JF, Dijk DJ, Klerman EB, et al. Later endogenous circadian temperature nadir relative to an earlier wake time in older people. Am J Physiol 1998;275:R1478–87.

20. Dijk DJ, Duffy JF, Czeisler CA. Age-related increase in awakenings: impaired consolidation of nonREM sleep at all circadian phases. Sleep 2001;24(5): 565–77.

21. Morgenthaler TI, Lee-Chiong T, Alessi C, et al. Practice parameters for the clinical evaluation and treatment of circadian rhythm sleep disorders. An American Academy of Sleep Medicine report. Sleep 2007;30(11):1445–59.

22. Rahman SA, Kayumov L, Tchmoutina EA, et al. Clinical efficacy of dim light melatonin onset testing in diagnosing delayed sleep phase syndrome. Sleep Med 2009;10(5):549–55.

23. Foley DJ, Monjan AA, Brown SL, et al. Sleep complaints among elderly persons: an epidemiologic study of three communities. Sleep 1995;18(6): 425–32.

24. Foley D, Ancoli-Israel S, Britz P, et al. Sleep disturbances and chronic disease in older adults: results of the 2003 National Sleep Foundation Sleep in America Survey. J Psychosom Res 2004;56(5): 497–502.

25. Sack RL, Auckley D, Auger RR, et al. Circadian rhythm sleep disorders: part II, advanced sleep phase disorder, delayed sleep phase disorder, free-running disorder, and irregular sleep-wake rhythm. An American Academy of Sleep Medicine review. Sleep 2007;30(11):1484–501.

26. Monk TH, Buysse DJ. Chronotype, bed timing and total sleep time in seniors. Chronobiol Int 2014; 31(5):655–9.

27. Uchiyama M, Lockley SW. Non-24-hour sleep-wake rhythm disorder in sighted and blind patients. Sleep Med Clin 2015;10(4):495–516.

28. Zee PC, Vitiello MV. Circadian rhythm sleep disorder: irregular sleep wake rhythm type. Sleep Med Clin 2009;4(2):213–8.

29. Ancoli-Israel S, Klauber MR, Jones DW, et al. Variations in circadian rhythms of activity, sleep, and light exposure related to dementia in nursing-home patients. Sleep 1997;20(1):18–23.

30. Sack RL, Auckley D, Auger RR, et al. Circadian rhythm sleep disorders: part I, basic principles, shift work and jet lag disorders. An American Academy of Sleep Medicine review. Sleep 2007;30(11):1460–83.

31. Duffy JF. Shift work and aging: roles of sleep and circadian rhythms. Clin Occup Environ Med 2003; 3:311–32.

32. Härmä M, Tenkanen L, Sjöblom T, et al. Combined effects of shift work and life-style on the prevalence of insomnia, sleep deprivation and daytime sleepiness. Scand J Work Environ Health 1998; 24:300–7.

33. Blackwell T, Yaffe K, Ancoli-Israel S, et al. Poor sleep is associated with impaired cognitive function in older women: the study of osteoporotic fractures. J Gerontol A Biol Sci Med Sci 2006;61(4):405–10.

34. Yaffe K, Blackwell T, Barnes DE, et al. Preclinical cognitive decline and subsequent sleep

disturbance in older women. Neurology 2007;69(3): 237–42.

35. Tranah GJ, Blackwell T, Ancoli-Israel S, et al. Circadian activity rhythms and mortality: the study of osteoporotic fractures. J Am Geriatr Soc 2010;58(2): 282–91.

36. Tranah GJ, Blackwell T, Stone KL, et al. Circadian activity rhythms and risk of incident dementia and mild cognitive impairment in older women. Ann Neurol 2011;70(5):722–32.

37. Lim AS, Yu L, Costa MD, et al. Increased fragmentation of rest-activity patterns is associated with a characteristic pattern of cognitive impairment in older individuals. Sleep 2012;35(5):633–640B.

38. Blackwell T, Yaffe K, Laffan A, et al. Associations of objectively and subjectively measured sleep quality with subsequent cognitive decline in older community-dwelling men: the MrOS sleep study. Sleep 2014;37(4):655–63.

39. Diem SJ, Blackwell TL, Stone KL, et al. Measures of sleep-wake patterns and risk of mild cognitive impairment or dementia in older women. Am J Geriatr Psychiatry 2016;24(3):248–58.

40. Kang JE, Lim MM, Bateman RJ, et al. Amyloid-beta dynamics are regulated by orexin and the sleep-wake cycle. Science 2009;326(5955): 1005–7.

41. Roh JH, Huang Y, Bero AW, et al. Disruption of the sleep-wake cycle and diurnal fluctuation of amyloid-B in mice with Alzheimer's disease pathology. Sci Transl Med 2012;4(150):1–10, 2013.

42. Xie L, Kang H, Xu Q, et al. Sleep drives metabolite clearance from the adult brain. Science 2013; 342(6156):373–7.

43. Van Someren EJ. Actigraphic monitoring of sleep and circadian rhythms. Handb Clin Neurol 2011; 98:55–63.

44. Oosterman JM, van Someren EJ, Vogels RL, et al. Fragmentation of the rest-activity rhythm correlates with age-related cognitive deficits. J Sleep Res 2009;18(1):129–35.

45. Wang JL, Lim AS, Chiang WY, et al. Suprachiasmatic neuron numbers and rest-activity circadian rhythms in older humans. Ann Neurol 2015;78(2): 317–22.

46. Satlin A, Volicer L, Stopa EG, et al. Circadian locomotor activity and core-body temperature rhythms in Alzheimer's disease. Neurobiol Aging 1995; 16(5):765–71.

47. Harper DG, Volicer L, Stopa EG, et al. Disturbance of endogenous circadian rhythm in aging and Alzheimer disease. Am J Geriatr Psychiatry 2005; 13(5):359–68.

48. Inouye SK, Marcantonio ER, Kosar CM, et al. The short-term and long-term relationship between delirium and cognitive trajectory in older surgical patients. Alzheimers Dement 2016;12(7):766–75.

49. Swaab DF, Fliers E, Partiman TS. The suprachiasmatic nucleus of the human brain in relation to sex, age and senile dementia. Brain Res 1985; 342:37–44.

50. Baloyannis SJ, Mavroudis I, Mitilineos D, et al. The hypothalamus in Alzheimer's disease: a Golgi and electron microscope study. Am J Alzheimers Dis Other Demen 2015;30(5):478–87.

51. Harper DG, Stopa EG, McKee AC, et al. Differential circadian rhythm disturbances in men with Alzheimer disease and frontotemporal degeneration. Arch Gen Psychiatry 2001;58(4): 353–60.

52. Gao L, Liu Y, Li X, et al. Abnormal retinal nerve fiber layer thickness and macula lutea in patients with mild cognitive impairment and Alzheimer's disease. Arch Gerontol Geriatr 2015;60(1):162–7.

53. Coppola G, Di Renzo A, Ziccardi L, et al. Optical coherence tomography in Alzheimer's disease: a meta-analysis. PLoS One 2015;10(8):e0134750.

54. La Morgia C, Ross-Cisneros FN, Koronyo Y, et al. Melanopsin retinal ganglion cell loss in Alzheimer disease. Ann Neurol 2016;79(1):90–109.

55. Chahine LM, Amara AW, Videnovic A. A systematic review of the literature on disorders of sleep and wakefulness in Parkinson's disease from 2005 to 2015. Sleep Med Rev 2017;35:33–50.

56. Videnovic A, Noble C, Reid KJ, et al. Circadian melatonin rhythm and excessive daytime sleepiness in Parkinson disease. JAMA Neurol 2014; 71(4):463–9.

57. Bordet R, Devos D, Brique S, et al. Study of circadian melatonin secretion pattern at different stages of Parkinson's disease. Clin Neuropharmacol 2003; 26(2):65–72.

58. Walsh CM, Ruoff L, Varbel J, et al. Rest-activity rhythm disruption in progressive supranuclear palsy. Sleep Med 2016;22:50–6.

59. Aziz NA, Pijl H, Frolich M, et al. Delayed onset of the diurnal melatonin rise in patients with Huntington's disease. J Neurol 2009;256(12):1961–5.

60. Morton AJ, Rudiger SR, Wood NI, et al. Early and progressive circadian abnormalities in Huntington's disease sheep are unmasked by social environment. Hum Mol Genet 2014;23(13):3375–83.

61. van Wamelen DJ, Aziz NA, Anink JJ, et al. Suprachiasmatic nucleus neuropeptide expression in patients with Huntington's disease. Sleep 2013;36(1): 117–25.

62. Czeisler CA, Allan JS, Strogatz SH, et al. Bright light resets the human circadian pacemaker independent of the timing of the sleep-wake cycle. Science 1986; 233:667–71.

63. Duffy JF, Zeitzer JM, Czeisler CA. Decreased sensitivity to phase-delaying effects of moderate intensity light in older subjects. Neurobiol Aging 2007;28: 799–807.

64. Kim SJ, Benloucif S, Reid KJ, et al. Phase-shifting response to light in older adults. J Physiol 2014; 592(Pt 1):189–202.

65. Benloucif S, Green K, L'Hermite-Baleriaux M, et al. Responsiveness of the aging circadian clock to light. Neurobiol Aging 2006;27(12):1870–9.

66. Klerman EB, Duffy JF, Dijk DJ, et al. Circadian phase resetting in older people by ocular bright light exposure. J Investig Med 2001;49:30–40.

67. Khalsa SBS, Jewett ME, Cajochen C, et al. A phase response curve to single bright light pulses in human subjects. J Physiol 2003;549(Pt 3):945–52.

68. Chang AM, Santhi N, St Hilaire M, et al. Human responses to bright light of different durations. J Physiol 2012;590(Pt 13):3103–12.

69. Dewan K, Benloucif S, Reid K, et al. Light-induced changes of the circadian clock of humans: increasing duration is more effective than increasing light intensity. Sleep 2011;34(5):593–9.

70. Najjar RP, Zeitzer JM. Temporal integration of light flashes by the human circadian system. J Clin Invest 2016;126(3):938–47.

71. Herljevic M, Middleton B, Thapan K, et al. Light-induced melatonin suppression: age-related reduction in response to short wavelength light. Exp Gerontol 2005;40(3):237–42.

72. Sletten TL, Revell VL, Middleton B, et al. Age-related changes in acute and phase-advancing responses to monochromatic light. J Biol Rhythms 2009;24(1): 73–84.

73. Kessel L, Siganos G, Jorgensen T, et al. Sleep disturbances are related to decreased transmission of blue light to the retina caused by lens yellowing. Sleep 2011;34(9):1215–9.

74. Campbell SS, Dawson D, Anderson MW. Alleviation of sleep maintenance insomnia with timed exposure to bright light. J Am Geriatr Soc 1993;41: 829–36.

75. Suhner AG, Murphy PJ, Campbell SS. Failure of timed bright light exposure to alleviate age-related sleep maintenance insomnia. J Am Geriatr Soc 2002;50:617–23.

76. Pallesen S, Nordhus IH, Skelton SH, et al. Bright light treatment has limited effect in subjects over 55 years with mild early morning awakening. Percept Mot Skills 2005;101(3):759–70.

77. Auger RR, Burgess HJ, Emens JS, et al. Clinical practice guideline for the treatment of intrinsic circadian rhythm sleep-wake disorders: advanced sleep-wake phase disorder (ASWPD), delayed sleep-wake phase disorder (DSWPD), non-24-hour sleep-wake rhythm disorder (N24SWD), and irregular sleep-wake rhythm disorder (ISWRD). An update for 2015: an American Academy of Sleep Medicine Clinical Practice Guideline. J Clin Sleep Med 2015;11(10): 1199–236.

78. Pollak CP, Perlick D. Sleep problems and institutionalization of the elderly. J Geriatr Psychiatry Neurol 1991;4:204–10.

79. Pollak CP, Perlick D, Linsner JP, et al. Sleep problems in the community elderly as predictors of death and nursing home placement. J Community Health 1990;15(2):123–35.

80. Mishima K, Okawa M, Hishikaa Y, et al. Morning bright light therapy for sleep and behaviour disorders in elderly patients with dementia. Acta Psychiatr Scand 1994;89:1–7.

81. Satlin A, Volicer L, Ross V, et al. Bright light treatment of behavioral and sleep disturbances in patients with Alzheimer's disease. Am J Psychiatry 1992; 149:1028–32.

82. Ancoli-Israel S, Martin JL, Gehrman P, et al. Effect of light on agitation in institutionalized patients with severe Alzheimer disease. Am J Geriatr Psychiatry 2003;11(2):194–203.

83. Dowling GA, Burr RL, Van Someren EJ, et al. Melatonin and bright-light treatment for rest-activity disruption in institutionalized patients with Alzheimer's disease. J Am Geriatr Soc 2008;56(2): 239–46.

84. Riemersma-van der Lek RF, Swaab DF, Twisk J, et al. Effect of bright light and melatonin on cognitive and noncognitive function in elderly residents of group care facilities: a randomized controlled trial. J Am Med Assoc 2008;299(22):2642–55.

85. Figueiro MG, Plitnick BA, Lok A, et al. Tailored lighting intervention improves measures of sleep, depression, and agitation in persons with Alzheimer's disease and related dementia living in long-term care facilities. Clin Interv Aging 2014;9: 1527–37.

86. Alessi CA, Martin JL, Webber AP, et al. Randomized, controlled trial of a nonpharmacological intervention to improve abnormal sleep/wake patterns in nursing home residents. J Am Geriatr Soc 2005; 53(5):803–10.

87. Clendon J, Walker L. Nurses aged over 50 years and their experiences of shift work. J Nurs Manag 2013; 21(7):903–13.

88. Richter K, Acker J, Adam S, et al. Prevention of fatigue and insomnia in shift workers–a review of non-pharmacological measures. EPMA J 2016;7:16.

89. Crowley SJ, Lee C, Tseng CY, et al. Combinations of bright light, scheduled dark, sunglasses, and melatonin to facilitate circadian entrainment to night shift work. J Biol Rhythms 2003;18(6):513–23.

90. Walsh JK, Muehlbach MJ, Schweitzer PK. Hypnotics and caffeine as countermeasures for shiftwork-related sleepiness and sleep disturbance. J Sleep Res 1995;4(Suppl. 2):80–3.

91. Chinoy ED, Harris MP, Kim MJ, et al. Scheduled evening sleep and enhanced lighting improve

adaptation to night shift work in older adults. Occup Environ Med 2016;73(12):869–76.

92. Karoly L, Panis C. Shifting demographic patterns shaping the future workforce. The 21st century at work: forces shaping the future workforce and workplace in the United States. Santa Monica (CA): RAND Corporation; 2004.

93. Fung CH, Vitiello MV, Alessi CA, et al. Report and research agenda of the American Geriatrics Society and National Institute on Aging Bedside-to-Bench Conference on Sleep, Circadian Rhythms, and Aging: new avenues for improving brain health, physical health, and functioning. J Am Geriatr Soc 2016;64(12):e238–47.

Parasomnias and Sleep-Related Movement Disorders in Older Adults

Alex Iranzo, MD

KEYWORDS

- Sleep paralysis • Disorders of arousal • Idiopathic REM sleep behavior disorder
- Anti-IgLON5 disease • Restless legs syndrome • Periodic limb movement disorder

KEY POINTS

- Sleepwalking and night terrors may persist in the older adult.
- Zolpidem may induce sleepwalking and sleep-related eating.
- Patients with idiopathic rapid eye movement (REM) sleep behavior disorder (RBD) represent the prodromal stage of Parkinson disease and related synucleinopathies, and should be enrolled in disease-modifying trials.
- Anti-IgLON5 disease is characterized by abnormal sleep architecture, abnormal behaviors in NREM sleep, RBD, antibodies against the protein IgLON5, HLA-DQB1*05:01, and tau deposits involving the brainstem and the hypothalamus.
- Patients with a severe form of periodic limb movements in sleep involving the whole body may present with dream-enacting behaviors and unpleasant dreams.

INTRODUCTION

Parasomnias are undesirable physical events or experiences that occur during entry into sleep, within sleep, or during arousal from sleep.[1] Parasomnias may occur during rapid eye movement (REM) sleep, non-REM (NREM) sleep, or during transitions from and to sleep.[1] In this article, we review the parasomnias and other sleep-related disorders that can occur in older people.

SLEEP PARALYSIS

Sleep paralysis is the inability to perform voluntary movements at sleep onset or when waking from sleep, with a duration ranging from seconds to a few minutes.[1] Individuals experience sleep paralysis as an unpleasant phenomenon where they are completely aware that they cannot move, open their eyes, or speak that is usually linked to the feeling of suffocation, chest pressure, and, in extreme cases, the fear of dying. The events end abruptly and spontaneously or after tactile stimulation. The association with vivid visual, auditory, and tactile hallucinations is common. Sleep paralysis represents a dissociative state where REM sleep atonia coexists with the full consciousness of wakefulness. Sleep deprivation and an irregular sleep–wake schedule are predisposing factors. Sleep paralysis is common among healthy people with a prevalence of 15% to 40% of at least 1 episode, with onset usually in adolescence. Episodes may be recurrent and some subjects report a familial aggregation of the phenomenon. Sleep paralysis is very common in adolescents and young adults. However, in a few cases sleep paralysis may persist in older adults, particularly in families suffering from this phenomenon. In the

Disclosure Statement: The author has no disclosures regarding the topic covered in this article.
Neurology Service, Multidisciplinary Sleep Unit, Hospital Clinic de Barcelona, C/ Villarroel 180, Barcelona 08036, Spain
E-mail address: AIRANZO@clinic.cat

Sleep Med Clin 13 (2018) 51–61
https://doi.org/10.1016/j.jsmc.2017.09.005

sleep.theclinics.com

majority of cases, including those occurring in older adults, small doses of REM sleep suppressants such as clomipramine can reduce dramatically the frequency and intensity of the episodes.

DISORDERS OF AROUSALS

Disorders of arousal are parasomnias occurring in NREM sleep and comprise confusional arousals, sleepwalking, and sleep terrors. Clinically, patients present with brief recurrent episodes of confused, complex, and bizarre behaviors; frightening screams; and walking. These symptoms arise as a result of incomplete and partial awakenings from deep sleep. Most of the cases are benign and idiopathic. A familial pattern is common, but a genetic signature has not been found. A positive correlation with the HLA-DQB1*05 subtype has been reported.[2,3] In contrast with popular belief, individuals with sleepwalking and sleep terrors usually have nightmares that are related to aggression, misfortune, and apprehension, and their sleep behaviors seem to involve fear and unpleasant confusion.[4] In severe cases, episodes may result in interrupted sleep, daytime fatigue, psychological problems, social effects, injuries, and medicolegal issues. Predisposing factors are those that result in deepened sleep (eg, sleep deprivation, night shifts, fever) and in sleep fragmentation (eg, noise, touch, psychological stress). Alcohol is another trigger.[4] Obstructive sleep apnea and periodic leg movements in sleep are not associated with disorders of arousals, but they can coexist by chance and then trigger some events when apneic episodes and limb movements cause arousals.

Disorders of arousal usually start during childhood, but can persist into adulthood up to the age of 60 years; they can also arise de novo in adulthood.[5] When disorders of arousal start in adulthood or older age, one has to suspect the effect of a medication (such as zolpidem) as the cause.

Disorders of arousal have been related to the effects of some medications. In most reports the disorder of arousal has not been documented by polysomnography (PSG). The assumption of drug-induced sleepwalking is based on the temporal association between the introduction of the drug and the onset of the abnormal sleep behaviors and their cessation after the drug is stopped. The most common drugs inducing sleepwalking are zolpidem (used at therapeutic doses for insomnia) and sodium oxybate (at high doses within the normal range used for narcolepsy). Postmarketing studies of zolpidem reported sleepwalking among between 0.3% and 1.0% of

the patients taking this medication. Besides sleepwalking, zolpidem can also cause the sleepwalking variants of sleep-related eating disorder, sleep driving, and sleep sex (which can occur in the same patient). There are a few case reports and small series of other medications that have induced or precipitated disorders of arousals (mainly sleepwalking), such as lithium carbonate, typical and atypical neuroleptics, zaleplon, stimulants, antihistamines, antidepressants (including paroxetine, bupropion and reboxetine [not available in the United States]), sedative hypnotics, statins, and topiramate. These medications may disturb sleep architecture and precipitate some events in predisposed individuals with and without a past history of disorders of arousal. These medications usually induce sleepwalking and its variants, including eating with consumption of peculiar forms or combinations of food (sleep-related eating disorder), smoking (sleep smoking), driving (sleep driving), and having sex (sleep sex or sexsomnia).

RAPID EYE MOVEMENT SLEEP BEHAVIOR DISORDER

REM sleep behavior disorder (RBD) is a REM sleep parasomnia characterized by dream-enacting behaviors and nightmares linked to REM sleep without muscle atonia. Owing to its association with neurodegenerative disorders, RBD warrants particular attention in a discussion of parasomnias and sleep-related movement disorders in older adults. The diagnosis of RBD requires confirmation with video-PSG because other sleep disorders (eg, obstructive sleep apnea, periodic limb movement disorder, nocturnal frontal lobe epilepsy, and sleepwalking) may also present with nightmares and abnormal sleep behaviors. RBD can be classified into an idiopathic form (IRBD) and a secondary form. Available data indicate that most patients with IRBD will eventually be diagnosed with the neurodegenerative disorders Parkinson disease (PD), dementia with Lewy bodies (DLB), or multiple system atrophy (MSA).[6,7] Patients with IRBD represent the prodromal stage of these synucleinopathies. The secondary form of RBD is related to known neurodegenerative diseases, autoimmune diseases, focal structural lesions in the brainstem, and the use of some medications. Psychiatric disorders are not linked to RBD.[6,7] IRBD and RBD secondary to the synucleinopathies occur in people older than 50 years of age, usually between the ages of 60 and 75. Herein we review IRBD and RBD secondary to the synucleinopathies PD, MSA, and DLB.

Idiopathic Rapid Eye Movement Sleep Behavior Disorder

The diagnosis of IRBD requires a history of dream-enacting behaviors, video-PSG detection of REM sleep with increased muscular activity associated with abnormal behaviors, the absence of known neurodegenerative diseases, lack of motor and cognitive complaints, normal neurologic examination, normal brain MRI studies, and RBD not explained by a brain lesion (eg, stroke, demyelinating plaque, encephalitis) or by the introduction or withdrawal of any medication or substance (eg, antidepressants, beta-blockers).[1,6] In many patients with IRBD, subclinical abnormalities can be detected such as olfactory deficits, cognitive deficits on neuropsychological tests, and decreased dopamine transporter imaging in the striatum on functional neuroimaging. These findings suggest that, when IRBD is diagnosed, a neurodegenerative process is likely already widespread in the nervous system. Of these abnormalities, hyposmia, color vision impairment, substantia nigra hyperechogenicity, and decreased striatal dopamine transporter uptake identify those patients with IRBD who are at increased short-term risk (2.5–5.0 years) for being diagnosed with a synucleinopathy according to accepted clinical criteria.[8,9] Prospective studies have further shown that the echogenic size of the substantia nigra,[10] color vision, olfactory dysfunction,[9] and dysautonomic changes[11] remain stable over time. In contrast, dopamine transporter imaging shows progressive decline in striatal tracer uptake.[12] Thus, dopamine transporter imaging serves better as a marker of subclinical progression in IRBD. The same happens with cognitive testing that shows worsening in executive, visuospatial, and memory domains over time.[13]

It has been shown that PD, DLB, and MSA frequently develop in patients with IRBD who are followed at sleep centers. In the seminal study, Schenck and colleagues[14] found that parkinsonism developed in 11 of 29 subjects with IRBD (38%) nearly 4 years after the diagnosis of IRBD and almost 13 years after the onset of RBD. After 16 additional years of follow-up, 21 patients with IRBD (72.4%) from the original cohort were diagnosed with PD in 13 cases, DLB in 3, MSA in 2, unspecified dementia in 1, and Alzheimer disease (with autopsy-confirmed combined Alzheimer disease pathology plus Lewy pathology) in 2. Three subjects with IRBD were lost during the follow-up period.[15] In a second series, we reported that 20 of 44 patients with IRBD (45%) developed a neurologic disorder after a mean interval of 11.5 years estimated from RBD onset and after a mean follow-up of 5.1 years from the diagnosis of IRBD. Emerging disorders were PD in 9 patients (2 with associated dementia), DLB in 6, MSA with predominant cerebellar syndrome in 1, and mild cognitive impairment (MCI) in 4 in whom visuospatial dysfunction was prominent. The finding that patients who developed a disorder were those with longer follow-up suggested that the conversion rate (45%) could increase with the passage of time.[16] This was confirmed after 7 additional years of follow-up of this original cohort. We found that, after a median follow-up of 10.5 years, 82% were diagnosed with PD (n = 16), DLB (n = 14), MSA (n = 1), and MCI (n = 5). The estimated risk of defined neurodegenerative syndrome from the diagnosis of IRBD was 34.8% at 5 years, 73.4% at 10 years, and 92.5% at 14 years.[17] These findings, in a group of 44 individuals with long and close follow-up indicate that most subjects with IRBD develop a synucleinopathy with time.

Because additional patients with IRBD were diagnosed and followed in our sleep center, we aimed to confirm our initial observation in a larger cohort of subjects that comprised all the 174 consecutive IRBD cases diagnosed up to July 2013 in our sleep center. The risk of a defined neurodegenerative syndrome from the time of IRBD diagnosis was 33.1% at 5 years, 75.7% at 10 years, and 90.9% at 14 years. Emerging diagnoses (37.4%) were DLB in 29 subjects, PD in 22, MSA in 2, and MCI in 12. In 6 cases who were diagnosed with PD, DLB ,and MCI, neuropathologic examination disclosed neuronal loss and widespread Lewy-type pathology in the brain in each case.[18] Similar findings were observed in other series.[19–22] Perhaps the most relevant evidence that IRBD represents a neurodegenerative condition is that in vivo biopsy of the colon and submandibular gland shows deposits of synuclein in subjects with IRBD but not in controls.[23,24]

Taken together, IRBD is an optimal population to test disease-modifying strategies to stop the neurodegenerative disease and prevent the clinical appearance of the cardinal manifestations of the synucleinopathies, namely parkinsonism and dementia.

The Transition Between Idiopathic Rapid Eye Movement Sleep Behavior Disorder and Clinical Diagnosis of Parkinson Disease, Dementia With Lewy Bodies, and Multiple System Atrophy

PD has a prodromal period of several years where progressive neuronal loss occurs before parkinsonism becomes clinically manifest and the disease can be clinically diagnosed. Olfactory loss, depression, constipation, and RBD may be present during the prodromal period of PD.[25] It is thought that DLB and MSA have also a prodromal phase before the clinical onset of their cardinal symptoms that define the disease (eg, dementia, parkinsonism, dysautonomia and cerebellar syndrome). We reported the case of a 63-year-old man that presented with IRBD and a 10-year clinical follow-up showed the serial development of constipation, hyposmia, depression, and MCI. The patient died without clinical parkinsonism and without dementia, and a postmortem examination showed neuronal loss and Lewy bodies in the entire brainstem, including the substantia nigra, olfactory bulb, hippocampus, and limbic system, and synuclein aggregates in the peripheral autonomic nervous system.[26]

One study evaluated the presence of motor signs in patients with IRBD.[27] In those patients with IRBD that developed PD with time, voice and face akinesia occurred earliest (estimated prodromal interval of nearly 10 years) followed by rigidity (4.4 years), gait abnormalities (4.4 years), and limb bradykinesia (4.2 years). In another prospective study clinically following 44 patients with IRBD, 16 patients (13 men and 3 women) were diagnosed with PD.[17] The mean age at PD diagnosis was 75 years, the estimated RBD duration at the time of the diagnosis of PD was 13 years, and the interval between diagnosis of IRBD and diagnosis of PD was 5.5 years. Five patients with PD developed dementia. In these 5 patients, the median interval between diagnosis of PD and development of dementia was 6 years. Patients with IRBD seen at sleep centers who later develop PD present a progressive parkinsonian syndrome, where rigidity, bradykinesia, and masked facies are prominent. This rigid–akinetic syndrome responds to levodopa. Resting tremor is not usually the presenting sign but this may occur at later stages of the disease. In these subjects, constipation and self-reported loss of smell are common before the emergence of parkinsonian signs. In some patients, parkinsonism occurs in parallel with the onset of MCI.

In patients with IRBD who later develop DLB, the first presentation may be (1) severe acute episodes of agitation, hallucinations, and delirium after elective surgery (eg, knee, hip, abdominal) that resolve spontaneously or with small doses of neuroleptics after 1 or 2 weeks, (2) subacute episodes of paranoid delusions and visual hallucinations, (3) isolated visual hallucinations such as bugs running on the floor or the sensation of having someone or a shadow behind his or her back, or (4) MCI. MCI is an intermediate stage between normal cognitive function and dementia where individuals have cognitive complaints, objective cognitive deficits detected on neuropsychological tests, and activities of daily living are preserved. In the setting of IRBD, MCI can be considered an abnormal condition that evolves into DLB and sometimes into PD. This is supported by several findings. First, MCI occurs in nearly 20% of patients with untreated PD at the time of initial diagnosis, and predicts conversion to dementia. Second, most patients with IRBD seen in sleep centers who develop MCI are eventually diagnosed with DLB. Third, patients with IRBD who develop MCI but not dementia show markers of a synucleinopathy, such as decreased striatal dopamine transporter, hyperechogenicity of the substantia nigra, and hyposmia. Finally, in patients with MCI with comorbid RBD who later develop dementia, postmortem examination shows Lewy body pathology.[26]

In our cohort of 44 subjects with IRBD described, 14 were eventually diagnosed with DLB.[17] All 14 subjects diagnosed with DLB were men. In these subjects with DLB, recurrent visual hallucinations occurred in 13 (93%), parkinsonism in 11 (79%), and fluctuating cognition in 9 (65%). Dementia was preceded by a recognized period of MCI characterized by executive, visuospatial, and memory dysfunction. The median interval between the diagnosis of MCI and the diagnosis of DLB was 2 years. The median age at DLB diagnosis was 76 years, the median estimated RBD duration at the time of the diagnosis of DLB was 12 years, and the median interval between diagnosis of RBD with video-PSG and clinical diagnosis of DLB was 7 years.

In patients with IRBD who later developed MSA with cerebellar signs, brain MRI may show atrophy of the pons and cerebellum before the emergence of a cerebellar syndrome. In these patients, urinary problems and falls owing to cerebellar ataxia may be one of the initial manifestations of the disease. Nocturnal stridor may also occur before the appearance of parkinsonism or ataxia in MSA.

Rapid Eye Movement Sleep Behavior Disorder in Patients Already Diagnosed with Parkinson Disease

PD is a neurodegenerative disorder characterized by parkinsonism, neuronal loss, and Lewy bodies in the substantia nigra and many other central and peripheral structures of the nervous system. RBD is common among PD, because cell loss is common within the neuronal structures that regulate REM sleep atonia, namely the subcoeruleus nucleus and magnocellularis nucleus in the brainstem and the amygdala. RBD occurs in patients with PD whether treated or untreated with dopaminergic agents. RBD is more common in MSA (90%–100%) and DLB (50%–70%) than in PD (25%–58%). A type of RBD-related unpleasant dreams, dream-enacting behaviors, and PSG abnormalities are similar among sporadic PD, MSA, and IRBD.[28] RBD has also been described in small series involving other neurodegenerative disorders such as progressive supranuclear palsy and Machado-Joseph disease.

RBD occurs in 25% to 58% of patients with sporadic PD, antedating the onset of parkinsonism by several years in about 20% of those with RBD.[29–32] RBD may precede parkinsonism, or it may develop concurrently or after the onset of parkinsonism. RBD confirmed by PSG may also occur in patients with PD linked to Parkin 2 mutations, but in this condition RBD-related clinical manifestations are usually mild. RBD was not detected in 1 PARK 6 family, an autosomal-recessive disorder that manifests as early-onset PD with a particularly mild progression. RBD occurs in PD associated with LRRK2 G2019S mutations where parkinsonism onset precedes RBD onset.[33] One study showed that, in subjects with sporadic PD, the report of sleep-related falling out of bed was clinically suggestive of RBD.[34] In a study involving nondemented patients with PD with RBD, video-PSG analysis and bed partners' reports demonstrated alleviation of parkinsonism during elaborate and complex RBD episodes. Movements during RBD episodes were faster, stronger, and smoother than those seen when the PD patient was awake. In the same manner, speech during RBD was more intelligible, better articulated, and louder than during wakefulness.[31]

RBD in manifested PD is associated with cognitive impairment, the rigid–akinetic motor subtype, older age, male predominance, autonomic dysfunction, and an increased risk to develop dementia over time. This suggests that the presence of RBD in PD predicts development of widespread neuropathological changes in the brain. Most studies have shown that in patients with nondemented, nonhallucinating sporadic PD, the presence of RBD in PD is neither associated with hypersomnia, sleep benefit, sleep architecture disruption, olfactory dysfunction, or lower daily levodopa equivalent dose. When patients with sporadic PD exhibit RBD, this parasomnia precedes the onset of parkinsonism in 18% to 22% of the cases.

Rapid Eye Movement Sleep Behavior Disorder in Patients Already Diagnosed with Multiple System Atrophy

MSA is a neurodegenerative disease clinically characterized by parkinsonism, dysautonomia, and cerebellar syndrome in any combination. The majority of patients with MSA have RBD.[35–37] The finding that in MSA brainstem cell loss is consistently widespread and severe, and may explain the high prevalence of RBD in this disease. RBD is currently considered a red flag for the diagnosis of MSA. In 1 study, 21 consecutive patients with MSA without sleep behavioral complaints underwent video-PSG that demonstrated RBD in 19 (90.5%).[36] In another study, video-PSG showed RBD in 35 of 37 (95%) consecutive patients with MSA.[35]

Self-awareness of abnormal sleep behaviors and unpleasant dream recall is variable among MSA subjects with RBD. In 1 study, 27 of 39 consecutive patients with MSA (69%) with RBD or their relatives reported dream-enacting behaviors. Interestingly, most of the 12 that did not report dream-enacting behaviors were sleeping alone at their home.[35] In another study, only 7 of 21 patients with MSA with RBD (33%) recalled vivid dreams.[36] In our first published case series comprising 26 consecutive MSA cases with RBD free of psychoactive drugs, 77% of patients were unaware of their abnormal behaviors, which were only noticed by bed partners. Recall of unpleasant dreams was absent in 35% of the patients.[28] Like in PD, RBD-related movements are faster, stronger, and smoother than during wakefulness.[36]

RBD may be the first symptom of MSA.[38,39] In 1 study of 27 patients with RBD aware of their dream-enacting behaviors, RBD preceded the waking motor symptoms in 12 (44%).[36] In another study of 19 patients, RBD features were reported by the patients or their relatives as the first manifestation of the disease in 3, concomitant with other symptoms in 9, and developed after the onset of waking symptoms in the remaining 7 patients. In our series, RBD onset antedated parkinsonian, cerebellar, and dysautonomic onset in 35 of 67 patients (52%) by a mean of 7 years (range, 1–38).[28] MSA is eventually diagnosed in only a few subjects with the initial diagnosis of IRBD (most of them are diagnosed with PD and DLB), probably because in the general population MSA is much more rare than PD and DLB. We reported a patient presenting with dysautonomia, stridor during sleep, and RBD without parkinsonism or cerebellar syndrome in whom brain pathology disclosed MSA after sudden death during wakefulness.[38]

Rapid Eye Movement Sleep Behavior Disorder in Patients Already Diagnosed with Dementia with Lewy Bodies

DLB has been described as the second most common cause of neurodegenerative dementia after Alzheimer disease. It is characterized by parkinsonism, recurrent visual hallucinations, and fluctuations in cognition and alertness. DLB is diagnosed if dementia precedes or occurs within 1 year before the onset of parkinsonism. Neuronal loss and Lewy bodies are found in the brainstem, limbic system, and neocortex.[40]

The most studied sleep disturbance in DLB is RBD. Available data indicate that, in subjects with DLB, RBD is common, may be the first symptom of the disease, is associated with less Alzheimer disease pathology in the brain, and can be considered a red flag of the disease. RBD is very rare in Alzheimer disease and other forms of dementia, with the exception of PD associated with dementia. A retrospective study involving 37 consecutive patients with dementia plus RBD showed that 34 (92%) were male.[41] In 35 (96%), RBD symptoms preceded or occurred simultaneously with the cognitive complaints. The diagnosis of DLB was confirmed in the 3 patients that underwent autopsy and supported the notion that the combination of dementia and RBD most often reflects DLB. This finding is in agreement with neuropathologic studies in patients with antemortem diagnosis of DLB plus RBD showing cell loss and Lewy bodies in the brainstem, limbic system, and neocortex.[42,43] In a cohort of 234 autopsy-confirmed patients with dementia followed longitudinally, a history suggestive of RBD was present in 76% of 98 with autopsy-confirmed DLB, indicating that RBD is a common feature of DLB. In contrast, only 6 of the 136 patients without autopsy-confirmed DLB exhibited RBD.[43] Thus, inclusion of RBD improves the diagnostic accuracy of DLB. Dugger and colleagues[44] compared the clinical characteristics of 71 DLB patients with RBD and 19 without RBD. Those with RBD were predominantly male, had a shorter duration of dementia, an earlier onset of parkinsonism and visual hallucinations, and less Alzheimer disease-related pathology on autopsy. In 54 of the 71 patients with RBD (76%), this parasomnia coincided or developed before dementia onset. This group of patients in whom RBD developed before cognitive impairment were characterized by earlier onset of visual hallucinations and parkinsonism, more severe baseline parkinsonism and shorter duration of dementia.

In a retrospective study, Pao and colleagues[45] reviewed the polysomnographic findings of 78 DLB patients (71 male; mean age, 71 years) with sleep-related complaints. Seventy-5 patients (96%) had histories of dream-enactment behaviors with 65 (83%) showing confirmation of RBD during PSG. The remaining 13 subjects did not attain any REM sleep, and hence RBD could not be confirmed by PSG.

Terzaghi and colleagues[46] evaluated the clinical and video-PSG findings of 29 consecutive DLB patients. Patients were taking levodopa but no dopamine agonists, benzodiazepines, cholinergics, neuroleptics, or antidepressants. All 21 patients were male, their mean age was 75 years, and the mean disease duration was 3 years. Dissociated or ambiguous sleep was found in 6 patients who had severe dementia. Disruptive motor behaviors during sleep were found in 70% and consisted of RBD in 11 subjects, confusional episodes from NREM sleep in 7 cases, and arousal-related episodes from REM or NREM sleep mimicking RBD in 2.

Ferman and colleagues[47] evaluated (with PSG) 61 DLB patients with a mean estimated duration of cognitive impairment of 4 years and a mean estimated duration of RBD of 10 years. PSG showed REM sleep without atonia in 71% (of note, 19% of patients did not achieve REM sleep during PSG). Ratti and colleagues[48] evaluated (with PSG) a group of DLB patients and showed that those who reported sleep-related motor events corresponded either with RBD or with awakenings from sleep.

PARASOMNIA OVERLAP DISORDER

Parasomnia overlap disorder describes patients who have coexisting NREM sleep disorder of arousal and RBD. Parasomnia overlap disorder can be idiopathic or associated with conditions such as narcolepsy, Moebius syndrome (a rare neurologic condition with facial muscle weakness), and brain structural lesions.[49] The link between these 2 types of parasomnia can be by chance in a subject who had a disorder of arousal during childhood and decades later developed RBD. In some cases, this finding may explain subjects with IRBD who are greater than 60 years of age and report their abnormal behaviors started 30 to 50 years earlier. In contrast with IRBD, the risk of conversion to a neurodegenerative disease is unknown in parasomnia overlap disorder. This condition is rare and only a few cases have been confirmed by video-PSG. We reported video-PSG documentation of a patient with NREM parasomnia and normal REM sleep who, after several years of follow-up, developed RBD with persistence of NREM parasomnia.[50]

ANTI-IgLON5 DISEASE

The recently described anti-IgLON5 disease is a novel neurologic condition initially described in 8 unrelated older adults (median age at disease onset, 59 years; range, 52–76) in whom subacute

(2 cases) and chronic (6 cases) presentations were noted.[51] Patients presented clinically with witnessed apneic events, abnormal sleep behaviors, and additional waking neurologic symptoms such as gait instability, dysarthria, dysphagia, and mild dysautonomia. Patients had no previous history of disorders of arousal and were unaware of their sleep behaviors that were only noted by the bed partner. Video-PSG showed a very complex and novel sleep pattern characterized by (1) normal occipital alpha rhythm during wakefulness, (2) a slight reduction of total sleep time and sleep efficiency, (3) a distinctive temporal sequence of sleep stages and behaviors taking place, from most abnormal at the beginning of the night to normalization at the end, (4) infrequent normal N1 sleep and infrequent normal N2 sleep, (5) normal N3 sleep with delta waves only in the second half of the night, (6) initiation of sleep and re-entering of sleep after awakenings characterized by theta activity and rapid repetitive leg movements that do not fit criteria of periodic leg movements in sleep, (7) periods of diffuse delta activity, typical of normal N3 sleep, mixed with spindles, (8) poorly structured stage N2 sleep characterized by clear spindles and K complexes with frequent vocalizations (eg, talking, laughing, crying) simple motor activity (eg, raising the arm, punching) and finalistic behaviors (eg, goal-directed behaviors like sucking the thumbs while apparently eating, manipulating wires), (9) RBD, and (10) obstructive sleep apnea and inspiratory stridor secondary to vocal cord palsy. Longitudinal follow-up by video-PSG showed no dramatic deterioration of these sleep features with time. Autoantibodies against IgLON5, a neuronal cell adhesion protein, were identified in all patients. The haplotypes DQB1*0501 and DRB1*1001 were detected in all 4 patients tested. Most of the patients deceased after sudden death during wakefulness or at sleep. Neuropathology performed in 2 patients showed a tauopathy mainly involving the tegmentum of the brainstem and the hypothalamus.

After this initial publication, other patients were reported and neuropathologic criteria were established for this new entity.[52–59] A recent review of 22 patients revealed that the median age was 64 years (range, 46–83).[60] At the initial visit, 15 patients (68%) already complained of sleep symptoms. By the time of diagnosis of the disorder (median delay from symptom onset was 2.5 years, with a range of 2 months to 18 years), 4 clinical presentations were identified: (1) a predominant sleep disorder with NREM parasomnia and sleep breathing symptoms, (2) bulbar syndrome characterized by dysphagia, dysarthria, sialorrhea, and acute respiratory insufficiency, (3) a syndrome resembling progressive supranuclear palsy, and (4) cognitive impairment resembling Huntington disease. Reasons for referral were sleep disturbances in 8 patients, gait dysfunction in 8, and other symptoms in 6 (3 bulbar, 2 chorea, 1 cognitive decline). Thirteen of 15 patients (86.6%) had the HLA-DRB1*10:01 and HLA-DQB1*05:01 alleles. The risk ratio calculation indicated that DRB1*10:01 was 36 times more frequent in these patients than in the general population. Thirteen patients had IgLON5 antibodies in serum and the cerebrospinal fluid, and 2 only in serum. The disease was refractory to immunotherapy by the time of diagnosis, and postmortem findings were consistent with a novel neuronal tauopathy mainly involving the hypothalamus and tegmentum of the brainstem. It remains unclear if this condition is a neurodegenerative or an autoimmune disease.

RESTLESS LEGS SYNDROME

Restless legs syndrome (RLS) is a chronic sensorimotor entity that increases in prevalence with age in both genders, reaching a plateau in the sixth decade. RLS is characterized by an urge to move the legs, usually accompanied by unpleasant or uncomfortable sensations in the legs that begins or worsens during periods of rest or inactivity, such as lying or sitting. Typically, RLS starts in the evening or at night and is partially or totally relieved by movement such as walking, stretching, or stomping.[61] The unpleasant sensations are habitually felt deep inside the legs and most patients define them as a creepy and crawling sensation. Some patients, however, have difficulty finding a precise word or term to describe the abnormal sensations in their legs. Only a few patients describe the sensations in their legs as painful. RLS may involve 1 or both lower limbs and, in some cases, the symptoms spread to the upper limbs and, in severe cases, to the trunk, neck, and face. In the lower limbs, the legs are almost always affected, but it is not rare that the uncomfortable sensations reach the thighs and hips. Involvement of the feet is unusual, but it may occur. In the upper limbs, shoulders, arms, elbows, and forearms are more frequently affected than wrists and hands. In a few cases, RLS symptoms may occur exclusively in the abdomen or in other body parts. The time of RLS peak intensity is between 23:00 and 03:00, and nadir is in the morning between 06:00 and 10:00. Neurologic examination is usually normal except in those cases where RLS is secondary to varicose veins and/or polyneuropathy.

The clinical spectrum of RLS is wide, ranging from mild to severe forms. The severity of RLS depends on the frequency and intensity of both the urge to move and unpleasant sensations in the legs. Some cases have a progressive course, others have a stable course, and others present with unpredictable long fluctuations and remissions. In some individuals, RLS may be precipitated or aggravated by some specific circumstances including pregnancy, iron deficiency, and the introduction of certain medications such as antidepressants and antidopaminergics. Patients with mild RLS usually do not seek medical attention because symptoms are mild, sporadic, and not bothersome. Severe cases usually seen in medical practice may be associated with impaired general quality of life linked either to insomnia, sleep fragmentation, daytime sleepiness, depression, anxiety, fatigue, inability to concentrate, or social limitations (eg, inability to enjoy quiet activities at night that require sitting such as driving for a long time, traveling by plane, dining in a restaurant, or watching a movie in a theater).[61]

RLS may be sporadic, familial, or secondary to several conditions including end-stage renal disease, iron deficiency, pregnancy, some forms of peripheral neuropathy, and the use of antidopaminergic medications. RLS affects both sexes and all ages.[62] For unknown reasons, it is more frequent in women than in men. One study reported that experiencing RLS more than 4 nights per month occurred in 3% of participants aged 18 to 29 years, 10% of those aged 30 to 79 years, and 19% of those 80 years and older. About 20% of adults with RLS report onset of the symptoms between the ages of 10 and 20 years. A positive family history occurs in approximately 30% to 50% of the cases. In some cases, an autosomal-dominant mode of inheritance may be present. RLS is linked to some genetic variants in the BTBD9, MEIS1, and MAP2K5-LBXCOR1 genes.[63–65]

There is a growing body of literature that indicates that the pathophysiology of RLS is linked to decreased dopaminergic tone in the spinal cord and iron insufficiency in the brain.[66,67]

Dopaminergic agonists (pramipexole, ropinirole, and rotigotine) are considered the first line therapy for RLS.[68] However, in RLS, long-term therapy with dopaminergic agents may be related to a change in symptomatology termed augmentation.[69,70] The augmentation phenomenon is a complication which consists of (1) an overall increase of RLS symptom severity, (2) earlier onset of symptoms in the afternoon, (3) extension of the symptoms to previously unaffected body parts including the upper limbs, and (4) a shorter therapeutic effect of the dopaminergic medication. Management of the augmentation phenomenon includes decreasing the dose or withdrawal of the dopaminergic agent. Dopamine agonists may also induce impulse control disorders.

Nondopaminergic medications such as gabapentin, pregabalin, and oxycodone are also effective in the treatment of RLS. Iron replacement is necessary in cases with iron deficiency or when iron is normal but serum ferritin levels are low or in the lower normal range.[68,69]

PERIODIC LIMB MOVEMENTS IN SLEEP

Periodic limb movements in sleep (PLMS) are stereotyped repetitive movements characterized by dorsal flexion of the foot and sometimes flexion of the knee and even the hip in severe cases. The period length between 2 consecutive leg movements is 5 to 90 seconds. Each movement lasts between 0.5 and 10.0 seconds. PLMS occur in a series of at least 4 movements. They may occur in 1 or both legs.[71] PLMS occur in about 80% to 90% of cases of RLS. PLMS are also found in other disorders and in healthy individuals without motor, sensory, or sleep complains. In healthy subjects, the prevalence of PLMS increases with age. In healthy people older than 60 years without sleep complains, the mean number of PLMS is 25 per hour.[72] Thus, the absence of PLMS does not exclude RLS, and the presence of PLMS is not specific for RLS.

PLMS may be asymptomatic or may fragment sleep continuity leading to nonrestorative sleep. Periodic limb movement disorder refers to the situation where PLMS induce clinically significant sleep disturbance such as insomnia or hypersomnia.[1] We recently reported a new form of periodic limb movement disorder that is associated with vigorous limb and body movements and unpleasant dreams mimicking IRBD.[73] These individuals were 5 men and 2 women with a median age of 66 years who were evaluated because of abnormal sleep behaviors and nightmares resembling RBD. In these patients, video-PSG ruled out REM sleep parasomnia and showed frequent and vigorous PLMS in NREM sleep involving the 4 limbs and trunk and associated with semipurposeful behaviors and vocalizations occurring during arousals that followed these prominent PLMS. After treatment with dopaminergic agonists, PLMS were less frequent and vigorous, and unpleasant dreams and behaviors during sleep were dramatically improved. This form of severe PLMS should be considered as another condition that may simulate RBD symptoms and are part of the periodic limb movement disorder spectrum. Sleep specialists and neurologists should be aware of this entity in the differential diagnosis of RBD, and should consider video-PSG as the test able to distinguish RBD from this extreme form of PLMS or other entities (such as obstructive sleep apnea) that can mimic RBD symptoms.[74]

SUMMARY

Parasomnias and sleep-related movement disorders are important problems in older adults. Sleep paralysis is rare in older adults, but may occur in those with a family history of the condition. In addition, although uncommon, some patients with disorders of arousal (ie, confusional arousals, sleepwalking, sleep terrors) can have persistent symptoms into older age. Medications can also be the culprit in conditions such as sleepwalking and sleep-related eating, which can occur in older adults. RBD is an important condition in older adults, that warrants particular attention. Convincing longitudinal studies indicate that RBD represents a prodromal stage of Parkinson's disease, DLB and other synucleinopathies. In addition, anti-IgLON5 disease is a recently identified novel condition (that occurs in older adults) and includes abnormal behaviors in both NREM and REM sleep. RLS also remains an important condition to consider in older adults, given the increased prevalence with age. Finally, a severe form of PLMS may clinically mimic RBD. Clinicians should be aware of these important conditions, which can have a significant impact on the health and well-being of their older patients.

REFERENCES

1. American Academy of Sleep Medicine. International classification of sleep disorders. 3rd edition. Darien (IL): American Academy of Sleep Medicine; 2014.
2. Lecendreux M, Bassetti C, Dauvilliers Y, et al. HLA and genetic susceptibility to sleepwalking. Mol Psychiatry 2003;8:114–7.
3. Heidbreder A, Frauscher B, Mitterling T, et al. Not only sleepwalking but NREM parasomnia irrespective of the type is associated with HLA DQB1*05: 01. J Clin Sleep Med 2016;12:565–70.
4. Oudiette D, Leu S, Pottier M, et al. Dreamlike mentations during sleepwalking and sleep terrors in adults. Sleep 2009;32:1621–7.
5. Zadra A, Desautels A, Petit D, et al. Somnambulism: clinical aspects and pathophysiological hypothesis. Lancet Neurol 2013;12:285–94.
6. Iranzo A, Santamaria J, Tolosa E. Idiopathic rapid eye movement sleep behaviour disorder: diagnosis, management, and the need for neuroprotective interventions. Lancet Neurol 2016;15:405–19.
7. Boeve B. REM sleep behaviour disorder. Updated review of the core features, the REM sleep behaviour disorder-neurodegenerative disease association, evolving concepts, controversies, and future directions. Ann N Y Acad Sci 2010;1184:15–54.
8. Iranzo A, Lomeña F, Stockner H, et al, for the Sleep Innsbruck Barcelona (SINBAR) group. Decreased striatal dopamine transporter uptake and substantia nigra hyperechogenicity as risk markers of synucleinopathy in patients with idiopathic rapid-eye-movement sleep behaviour disorder: a prospective study. Lancet Neurol 2010;9:1070–7.
9. Postuma RB, Gagnon JF, Vendette M, et al. Olfaction and color vision identify impending neurodegeneration in rapid eye movement sleep behavior disorder. Ann Neurol 2011;69:811–8.
10. Iranzo A, Stockner H, Serradell M, et al. Five year follow-up of substantia nigra echogenecity in idiopathic REM sleep behavior disorder. Mov Disord 2014;29:1774–80.
11. Postuma RB, Gagnon JF, Vendette M, et al. Markers of neurodegeneration in idiopathic rapid eye movement sleep behavior disorder and Parkinson's disease. Brain 2009;13:3298–307.
12. Iranzo A, Valldeoriola F, Lomeña F, et al. Serial dopamine transporter imaging of nigrostriatal function in patients with idiopathic rapid-eye-movement sleep behaviour disorder: a prospective study. Lancet Neurol 2011;10:797–805.
13. Fantini ML, Farini E, Ortelli P. Longitudinal study of cognitive function in idiopathic REM sleep behavior disorder. Sleep 2011;34:619–25.
14. Schenck CH, Bundlie SR, Mahowald MW. Delayed emergence of a parkinsonian disorder in 38% of 29 older men initially diagnosed with idiopathic rapid eye movement sleep behavior disorder. Neurology 1996;46:388–92.
15. Schenck CH, Boeve BF, Mahowald MW. Delayed emergence of a parkinsonian disorder or dementia in 81% of older males initially diagnosed with idiopathic REM sleep behavior disorder (IRBD): 16 year update on a previously reported series. Sleep Med 2013;14:744–8.
16. Iranzo A, Molinuevo JL, Santamaria J, et al. Rapid-eye-movement sleep behaviour disorder as an early marker for a neurodegenerative disease: a descriptive study. Lancet Neurol 2006;5:572–7.
17. Iranzo A, Tolosa E, Gelpi E, et al. Neurodegenerative status and post-mortem pathology in idiopathic rapid-eye-movement disorder: an observational cohort study. Lancet Neurol 2013;12:443–53.
18. Iranzo A, Fernández-Arcos A, Tolosa E, et al. Neurodegenerative disorder risk in idiopathic REM sleep behavior disorder: study in 174 patients. PLoS One 2014;9(2):e89741.
19. Postuma RB, Gagnon JF, Bertrand JA, et al. Parkinson risk in idiopathic REM sleep behavior disorder: preparing for neuroprotective trials. Neurology 2015;84:1104–13.

20. Wing YK, Li SX, Mok V, et al. Prospective outcome of rapid eye movement sleep behaviour disorder: psychiatric disorders as a potential early marker of Parkinson's disease. J Neurol Neurosurg Psychiatry 2012;83:470–2.

21. Youn S, Kim T, Yoon IY, et al. Progression of cognitive impairments in idiopathic REM sleep behaviour disorder. J Neurol Neurosurg Psychiatry 2016; 87(8):890–6.

22. Postuma RB, Iranzo A, Hogl B, et al. Risk factors for neurodegeneration in idiopathic rapid eye movement sleep behavior disorder: a multicenter study. Ann Neurol 2015;77:830–9.

23. Sprenger FS, Stefanova N, Gelpi E, et al. Enteric nervous system α-synuclein immunoreactivity in idiopathic REM sleep behavior disorder. Neurology 2015;85:1761–8.

24. Vilas D, Iranzo A, Tolosa E, et al. Assessment of α-synuclein in submandibular glands of patients with idiopathic rapid-eye-movement sleep behaviour disorder: a case-control study. Lancet Neurol 2016;15: 708–18.

25. Tolosa E, Pont-Sunyer C. Progress in defining the premotor phase of Parkinson's disease. J Neurol Sci 2011;310:4–8.

26. Iranzo A, Gelpi E, Tolosa E, et al. Neuropathology of prodromal Lewy body disease. Mov Disord 2014;29: 410–5.

27. Postuma RN, Lang AE, Gagnon JF, et al. How does parkinsonism start? Prodromal parkinsonism motor changes in idiopathic REM sleep behaviour disorder. Brain 2012;27:617–26.

28. Iranzo A, Rye DB, Santamaria J, et al. Characteristics of idiopathic REM sleep behavior disorder and that associated with MSA and PD. Neurology 2005; 65:247–52.

29. Wetter TC, Trenkwalder C, Gershanik O, et al. Polysomnographic measures in Parkinson's disease: a comparison between patients with and without REM sleep disturbances. Wien Klin Wochenschr 2001;113:249–53.

30. Gagnon JF, Vendette M, Postuma R, et al. Mild cognitive impairment in rapid eye movement sleep behaviour disorder and Parkinson disease. Ann Neurol 2009;66:39–47.

31. De Cock VC, Vidailhet M, Leu S, et al. Restoration of normal motor control in Parkinson's disease during REM sleep. Brain 2007;130:450–6.

32. Sixel-Doring F, Trautmann E, Mollenhauer B, et al. Associated factors for REM sleep behaviour disorder in Parkinson disease. Neurology 2011;77:1048–54.

33. Pont-Sunyer C, Iranzo A, Gaig C, et al. Sleep disorders in parkinsonian and nonparkinsonian LRRK2 mutation carriers. PLoS One 2015;10(7):e0132368.

34. Wallace DM, Shafazand S, Carvalho DZ, et al. Sleep-related falling out of bed in Parkinson's disease. J Clin Neurol 2012;8:51–7.

35. Plazzi G, Corsini R, Provini F, et al. REM sleep behavior disorders in multiple system atrophy. Neurology 1997;48:1094–7.

36. De Cock V, Debs R, Oudiette D, et al. The improvement of movement of speech during rapid eye movement sleep behavior disorder in multiple system atrophy. Brain 2011;134:856–62.

37. Palma JA, Fernandez-Cordon C, Coon EA, et al. Prevalence of REM sleep behavior disorder in multiple system atrophy: a multicenter study and meta-analysis. Clin Auton Res 2015;25:69–75.

38. Gaig C, Iranzo A, Tolosa E, et al. Pathologically description of a non-motor variant of multiple system atrophy. J Neurol Neurosurg Psychiatry 2008;79: 1399–400.

39. Tachibana N, Kimura K, Kitajama K, et al. REM sleep motor dysfunction in multiple system atrophy: with special emphasis on sleep talk as its early clinical manifestation. J Neurol Neurosurg Psychiatry 1997; 63:678–81.

40. McKeith IG, Dickson DW, Lowe J, et al. Diagnosis and management of dementia with Lewy bodies. Third report of the DLB consortium. Neurology 2005;65:1863–72.

41. Boeve BF, Silber MH, Ferman TJ, et al. REM sleep behavior disorder and degenerative dementia. An association likely reflecting Lewy body disease. Neurology 1998;51:363–70.

42. Boeve BF, Silber MH, Parisi JE. Synucleinopathy pathology and REM sleep behavior disorder plus dementia or parkinsonism. Neurology 2003;61:40–5.

43. Ferman TJ, Boeve BF, Smith GE, et al. Inclusion of RBD improves the diagnostic classification of dementia with Lewy bodies. Neurology 2011;77: 875–82.

44. Dugger BN, Boeve BF, Murray ME, et al. Rapid eye movement sleep behavior disorder and subtypes in autopsy-confirmed dementia with Lewy bodies. Mov Disord 2012;27:72–8.

45. Pao WC, Boeve BF, Ferman TJ, et al. Polysomnographc findings in dementia with Lewy bodies. Neurologist 2013;19:1–6.

46. Terzaghi M, Arnaldi D, Rizzetti MC, et al. Analysis of video-polysomnographic sleep findings in dementia with Lewy bodies. Mov Disord 2013;28:1416–23.

47. Ferman TJ, Smith GE, Dickson DW, et al. Abnormal daytime sleepiness in dementia with Lewy bodies compared to Alzheimer's disease using the multiple sleep latency test. Alzheimers Res Ther 2014; 6(9):76.

48. Ratti PL, Terzaghi M, Minafra A, et al. REM and NREM sleep enactment behaviors in Parkinson's disease, Parkinson's disease dementia and dementia with Lewy bodies. Sleep Med 2012;13:926–32.

49. Dumitrascu O, Schenck CH, Applebee G, et al. Parasomnia overlap disorder: a distinct pathophysiological entity or a variant of rapid eye movement

sleep behavior disorder? A case series. Sleep Med 2013;14:1217–20.

50. Matos N, Iranzo A, Gaig C, et al. Video-polysomnographic documentation of non-rapid eye movement sleep parasomnia followed by rapid eye movement sleep behavior disorder: a parasomnia overlap disorder? Sleep Med 2016;23:46–8.

51. Sabater L, Gaig C, Gelpi E, et al. A novel non-rapid-eye movement and rapid-eye-movement parasomnia with sleep breathing disorder associated with antibodies to IgLON5: a case series, characterisation of the antigen, and post-mortem study. Lancet Neurol 2014;13:575–86.

52. Gelpi E, Höftberger R, Graus F, et al. Neuropathological criteria of anti-IgLON5-related tauopathy. Acta Neuropathol 2016;132:531–43.

53. Högl B, Heidbreder A, Santamaria J, et al. IgLON5 autoimmunity and abnormal behaviours during sleep. Lancet 2015;385:1590.

54. Simabukuro MM, Sabater L, Adoni T, et al. Sleep disorder, chorea, and dementia associated with IgLON5 antibodies. Neurol Neuroimmunol Neuroinflamm 2015;2:e136.

55. Montojo MT, Piren V, Benkhadra F, et al. Mimicking progressive supranuclear palsy and causing Tako-Tsubo syndrome: a case report on IgLON5 encephalopathy [abstract]. Mov Disord 2015;30(Suppl 1): 710.

56. Brüggemann N, Wandinger KP, Gaig C, et al. Dystonia, lower limb stiffness, and upward gaze palsy in a patient with IgLON5 antibodies. Mov Disord 2016; 31:762–4.

57. Schröder JB, Melzer N, Ruck T, et al. Isolated dysphagia as initial sign of anti-IgLON5 syndrome. Neurol Neuroimmunol Neuroinflamm 2016;4(1): e302.

58. Haitao R, Yingmai Y, Yan H, et al. Chorea and parkinsonism associated with autoantibodies to IgLON5 and responsive to immunotherapy. J Neuroimmunol 2016;300:9–10.

59. Zhang W, Niu N, Cui R. Serial 18F-FDG PET/CT findings in a patient with IgLON5 encephalopathy. Clin Nucl Med 2016;41:787–8.

60. Gaig C, Graus F, Compta Y, et al. Clinical manifestations of the anti-IgLON5 disease. Neurology 2017; 88(18):1736–43.

61. Allen RP, Picchietti DL, Garcia-Borreguero D, et al. Restless legs syndrome/Willis-Ekbom disease diagnostic criteria: updated International Restless Legs Syndrome Study Group (IRLSSG) consensus criteria–history, rationale, description, and significance. Sleep Med 2014;15:860–73.

62. Garcia-Borreguero D, Egatz R, Winkelmann J. Epidemiology of restless legs syndrome: the current status. Sleep Med Rev 2006;10:153–67.

63. Stefansson H, Rye D, Hicks A, et al. A genetic risk factor for periodic limb movements in sleep. N Engl J Med 2007;357:703–5.

64. Winkelmann J, Schormair P, Lichtner P, et al. Genome-wide association study of restless legs syndrome identifies common variants in three genomic regions. Nat Genet 2007;39:1000–6.

65. Winkelmann J, Schormair B, Xiong L, et al. Genetics of restless legs syndrome. Sleep Med 2016. https://doi.org/10.1016/j.sleep.2016.10.012.

66. Rye DB. Parkinson's disease and RLS: the dopaminergic bridge. Sleep Med 2004;5:317–28.

67. Paulus W, Trenkwalder C. Less is more: pathophysiology of dopaminergic-therapy-related augmentation in restless legs syndrome. Lancet Neurol 2006; 10:878–86.

68. Winkelman JW, Armstrong MJ, Allen RP, et al. Practice guideline summary: treatment of restless legs syndrome in adults: report of the Guideline Development, Dissemination, and Implementation Subcommittee of the American Academy of Neurology. Neurology 2016;87:2585–93.

69. Garcia-Borreguero D, Silber MH, Winkelman JW, et al. Guidelines for the first-line treatment of restless legs syndrome/Willis-Ekbom disease, prevention and treatment of dopaminergic augmentation: a combined task force of the IRLSSG, EURLSSG, and the RLS-foundation. Sleep Med 2016;21:1–11.

70. García-Borreguero D. Dopaminergic augmentation in restless legs Syndrome/Willis-Ekbom disease: identification and management. Sleep Med Clin 2015;10:287–92.

71. Iber C, Ancoli-Israel S, Chesson A, et al, for the American Academy of Sleep Medicine. The AASM manual for the scoring of sleep and associated events: rules, terminology and technical specifications. 1st edition. Westchester (IL): American Academy of Sleep Medicine; 2007.

72. Pennestri MH, Whittom S, Adam B, et al. PLMS and PLMW in healthy subjects as a function of age: prevalence and interval distribution. Sleep 2006;29: 1183–7.

73. Gaig C, Iranzo A, Pujo M, et al. Periodic limb movements during sleep mimicking REM sleep behavior disorder. Sleep 2017;40(3). https://doi.org/10.1093/sleep/zsw063.

74. Iranzo A, Santamaría J. Severe obstructive sleep apnea mimicking REM sleep behavior disorder. Sleep 2005;28:203–6.

Neurodegenerative Disorders and Sleep

Raman K. Malhotra, MD

KEYWORDS

- Parkinson disease • Alzheimer disease • Dementia • Rapid eye movement sleep behavior disorder
- Sleep apnea • Insomnia • Circadian rhythm disorder • Restless legs syndrome

KEY POINTS

- Sleep disorders are common in neurodegenerative conditions.
- Certain sleep disorders are more common in specific neurodegenerative conditions. REM sleep behavior disorder is more commonly seen in Parkinson disease than in Alzheimer disease.
- Common sleep disorders that may occur in most neurodegenerative conditions include insomnia, sleep apnea, restless legs syndrome, and circadian rhythm disorders.

INTRODUCTION

Cerebral neurodegenerative disorders, such as Parkinson disease (PD) and dementia, are increasing in prevalence as the population ages. These disorders are characterized by neuronal cell loss and abnormal accumulation of protein in cells of the brain. Symptoms, such as tremor, muscle rigidity, imbalance, and impaired cognition, progressively worsen with time. Not only are there challenges in managing the primary symptoms of these conditions, but many of these patients also suffer from sleep complaints, such as insomnia or hypersomnia. Others may suffer from abnormal movements during sleep, known as rapid eye movement (REM) sleep behavior disorder (RBD). This disorder may be dangerous and disruptive to sleep, and can sometimes precede the development of other symptoms of neurodegenerative disorders by years or even decades. High rates of sleep disorders, such as insomnia, hypersomnia, sleep apnea, restless legs syndrome (RLS), and circadian rhythm disorders, in older adults with neurodegenerative disorders are likely caused by the underlying symptoms of the disease along with damage to sleep-controlling regions of the brain. It is important to recognize and properly manage these sleep disorders because treatment may improve symptoms of the neurodegenerative condition and improve quality of life.

PARKINSON DISEASE AND OTHER SYNUCLEINOPATHIES

PD is a progressive neurodegenerative condition that causes motor symptoms of bradykinesia, shuffling gait, tremor, and rigidity. It is the second most common neurodegenerative condition affecting more than 1% of the population older than 60 years of age.[1] Patients commonly present with postural instability and falls. The pathologic hallmark of PD is Lewy bodies, which are intraneuronal α-synuclein inclusions. Lewy bodies first involve lower brainstem areas before spreading next to the substantia nigra and eventually areas throughout the brain. Motor symptoms of PD typically respond well to dopamine therapy early in the course of the disease. There are a variety of nonmotor symptoms of PD, including autonomic, olfactory, and mood dysfunction, and poor sleep. Sleep disorders are seen in most patients with PD.[2] The most common sleep disorders are

Disclosure Statement: The author has no relevant disclosures, nor any financial or commercial conflicts of interest.
Department of Neurology, Saint Louis University School of Medicine, Monteleone Hall, 1438 South Grand Boulevard, St Louis, MO 63104, USA
E-mail address: Ramanmalhotramd@gmail.com

Sleep Med Clin 13 (2018) 63–70
https://doi.org/10.1016/j.jsmc.2017.09.006

insomnia, periodic limb movement disorder, sleep-disordered breathing, and RBD. In addition to PD, other synucleinopathies (which are central nervous system degenerative conditions caused by abnormal α-synuclein accumulation) include Lewy body dementia and multiple system atrophy, which are also associated with high rates of the same sleep disorders typically seen in patients with PD.

Sleep is disrupted in PD and other synucleinopathies for numerous reasons. The motor and nonmotor symptoms described previously can lead to poor sleep at night. Many medications used for PD can have side effects of sleepiness and poor sleep. In addition, the sleep-controlling centers of the brain are also affected by the underlying neurodegenerative process in the brain. Involvement of the pedunculopontine nucleus, locus ceruleus, pontine ceruleus alpha nucleus, and raphe nuclei are implicated in disorders of REM sleep and slow wave sleep, and have been directly localized as areas of involvement in some animal models of PD.[3]

Insomnia

Insomnia is defined by a complaint of repeated difficulties with initiating sleep, maintaining sleep, or waking up earlier than desired that occurs despite adequate time and opportunity for sleep. The symptoms should result in some form of daytime impairment to meet criteria for this disorder.[4] Patients suffering from synucleinopathies, such as PD, commonly complain of insomnia. Patients with PD more commonly suffer from sleep maintenance insomnia as compared with sleep-onset insomnia. One study cites sleep problems in 60% of patients with PD, with 76% complaining of poor sleep.[2] Insomnia may occur from a variety of issues (Box 1). The motor symptoms of PD can

---

Box 1
Common causes of insomnia in Parkinson disease

Motor symptoms (cramps, stiffness, impaired turning in bed)

Nocturia

Depression and/or anxiety

Medication side effect

Inadequate sleep hygiene

Restless legs syndrome

Sleep apnea

Circadian rhythm disorders

---

cause issues with muscle cramps, stiffness, and difficulties with turning or rolling in bed. Nonmotor symptoms, such as autonomic dysfunction (which can lead to frequent nocturia) or mood disorders, also contribute to sleep disruption. Many medications used for PD can cause disrupted sleep at night or sleepiness during the daytime (causing less sleepiness overnight). Sleep-controlling areas of the brain may be damaged leading to insomnia. As the PD and nervous system degeneration progresses, insomnia also worsens in incidence and severity. Underlying mood disorders and worsening motor and nonmotor PD symptoms also contribute to worse insomnia later in the course of the disease. Polysomnography in patients with PD demonstrates prolonged sleep latency and fragmented sleep with reduced slow wave sleep and REM sleep. Insomnia may often result in subjective complaints of daytime fatigue, irritability, mood changes, poor attention, trouble with motor skills, and may result in decreased ability to function at baseline during waking hours.

Diagnosis and evaluation of insomnia typically involves a good history of sleep habits, bedtimes, wake times, naps, and awakenings at night. Directed questions in regards to causes or exacerbating factors of insomnia, such as RLS, medications, motor symptoms of PD, sleep apnea, and circadian rhythm disorders, should be performed. Sleep logs, diaries, and sleep trackers, such as actigraphy or wearable devices, are helpful. Polysomnography may be necessary if insomnia is thought to be secondary to sleep apnea, periodic limb movement disorder, or parasomnias.

Management of insomnia includes identifying and addressing any underlying primary sleep disorders. In addition, good sleep habits and hygiene should be encouraged. Medications and their timing should be scrutinized and possibly altered. If motor symptoms of PD are keeping the patient up at night, dopamine therapy at night may be necessary to alleviate the symptoms to help induce and maintain sleep. Short-acting carbidopa/levodopa, long-acting carbidopa/levodopa, dopamine agonists, and transdermal dopamine (ie, rotigotine patch) have shown small benefits in motor symptoms during the night in small trials.[5] Sometimes the dopamine agent itself may be causing insomnia. A decrease in dose or change in timing of the doses may improve sleep.

Primary sleep disorders, such as RLS and circadian rhythm disturbances, need to be correctly identified as a cause of insomnia in patients with PD. RLS is seen in 15% to 20% of patients with PD.[6] RLS is difficult to distinguish from other causes of leg pain in this population, such as muscle spasms and arthritis. Serum ferritin and iron studies should be evaluated in these patients and replaced if low (ie, ferritin <50). Other treatments for RLS include dopamine agonists, gabapentin, pregabalin, and opioids. Some patients who present with sleep maintenance insomnia or early morning awakenings may have a circadian rhythm disorder, such as advanced sleep-wake phase disorder. This condition is seen more commonly in the older population and in patients with neurodegenerative disorders. Delayed sleep-wake phase disorder is also seen in this population and may present with sleep-onset insomnia or difficulties awakening in the morning. Circadian rhythm disturbances have been described in patients with PD, including disruption of circadian markers, such as cortisol and melatonin levels.[7,8] Diagnosis should include a detailed history, sleep logs, and actigraphy. Patients with advanced sleep-wake phase disorder demonstrate evening sleepiness with difficulties in staying asleep. A prolonged sleep latency and later wake times are commonly reported in delayed sleep-wake phase disorder. Treatment of advanced sleep-wake phase disorder involves evening bright light therapy. Treatment of delayed sleep-wake phase disorder involves bright light on awakening in the morning along with evening melatonin several hours before desired bedtime.

Hypnotic medications should be used judiciously in this population because of concerns of causing falls, worsened balance, and impaired cognition. Potential benefits of therapies should be weighed against their risks. Hypnotics used in the general adult populations are the same agents typically used in patients with PD. There are limited studies evaluating use in this specific population. Studies have demonstrated effectiveness of eszopiclone and another with doxepin in improving subjective impression of sleep in patients with PD, but not objective measurements.[9,10] Sedating antidepressants have been used, but there should be caution because they may worsen RLS or periodic limb movements of sleep. As in the general population, cognitive behavioral therapy for insomnia is strongly suggested as first-line therapy for treatment of insomnia, although again evidence is scarce in relation to its effectiveness specifically in patients with PD.

Hypersomnia

Excessive daytime sleepiness is a common symptom in patients with PD. Because hypersomnia is a side effect of dopamine therapy, this may present early on in the disease process when dopamine therapy is initiated for motor symptoms.[11] However, this is not the only reason that excessive daytime sleepiness may present in this population (Box 2). Many wake-promoting regions in the brain are affected in PD, including the locus coeruleus, raphe nucleus, and hypocretin neurons, among other areas. One study suggests that hypersomnia precedes the development of other motor symptoms in PD, demonstrating sleepy adults had a three times higher risk of developing PD than nonsleepy adults.[12] Sleepiness may present with sleep attacks, or sudden onset sleep, which are more commonly reported in patients with PD (up to 14%) than age-matched control subjects.[13] Sleep attacks are dangerous if they occur during driving, work, or other activities where a sudden change in alertness may be dangerous. Sleep attacks can also be a side effect of dopamine agonists commonly used as treatment in patients with PD. In PD and multiple system atrophy, there has been evidence of damage to hypocretin neurons in the hypothalamus, leading to a narcolepsy-like condition with related symptoms.[14] Low hypocretin levels have been measured in patients with PD with these symptoms.[15]

A careful interview and evaluation for primary sleep disorders (eg, sleep apnea, restless legs, insomnia) is an important first step. Sleepiness as a possible side effect of dopamine therapy must also be recognized in patients with PD presenting with hypersomnia. If these factors and other causes of hypersomnia have been addressed, then use of a wake-promoting agent can be considered. Agents used to treat hypersomnia and narcolepsy in the general population are the same ones used in patients with PD with hypersomnia. Caffeine, modafinil, and methylphenidate have all been shown to improve sleepiness in patients with PD.[16,17] One trial used sodium oxybate and demonstrated improvement in symptoms.[18] Given the age of the population, caution must be used when starting wake-promoting agents in patients with comorbid cardiac or

---

Box 2
Common causes of hypersomnia in Parkinson disease

Sleep apnea

Medication side effect

Loss of hypocretin neurons (central nervous system hypersomnia)

Insufficient sleep

Circadian rhythm disorder

REM sleep behavior disorder

psychiatric disorders, and adverse effects, such as hypertension, confusion, and agitation, should be monitored.

Sleep-Disordered Breathing

Sleep-disordered breathing in the form of central and obstructive sleep apnea is seen in a greater proportion of patients with PD than in age-matched control subjects, although some studies dispute this finding.[19] Polysomnography is the proper diagnostic test in this population, because typically there is also concern for RBD and periodic limb movement disorder, both of which are not able to be identified with home sleep apnea testing. A randomized placebo-controlled cross-over study of patients with PD showed improvements in sleep architecture and objective measures in sleepiness in the patients treated with continuous positive airway pressure (CPAP).[20] As in the general population, positive airway pressure is typically effective in treating obstructive sleep apnea, but adherence remains a glaring challenge. Use of CPAP in patients with multiple system atrophy demonstrated that more than 66% discontinued CPAP after a year in one study.[21] In addition to typical obstructive sleep apnea symptoms, patients with multiple system atrophy may present with stridor and laryngeal dysfunction, which is a poor prognostic factor and requires treatment with positive airway pressure or other forms of nocturnal ventilation.[22]

Parasomnias

Patients with PD may complain of abnormal movements during sleep. This may be from a variety of conditions including sleep myoclonus, periodic limb movements of sleep, tremor, dystonia, or parasomnias. RBD is the most common parasomnia seen in patients with PD, seen in up to 60% of patients with PD. RBD is even more common in multiple-system atrophy and Lewy body dementia (75% or higher).[23] RBD involves repeated episodes of sleep-related vocalization and/or complex motor behaviors that occur during REM sleep. Motor activity can be reaching, grabbing, kicking, or other vigorous motor activity that could lead to injury of the patient or bed partner.[4] Nonviolent behaviors, such as smiling, laughing, or shouting, can also occur. The patient does not typically ambulate, with almost all motor activity occurring in or next to the bed. Eyes are typically closed and the patient does not interact with the environment. If awoken from the event, the patient returns to normal levels of consciousness, but may remember dream content related to the motor activity. Patients with PD with RBD have fewer tremors, more falls, more autonomic dysfunction, and more cognitive dysfunction than patients with PD who do not have RBD.[24] RBD has been shown to be a prodromal stage for PD and other synucleinopathies. Studies following patients with idiopathic RBD have demonstrated high rates of conversion to PD and other synucleinopathies, with a 45% rate of conversion at 5 years, 76% rate at 10 years, and more than 90% rate at 14 years.[25] These patients with RBD at high risk for central nervous degenerative disorders will likely be ideal candidates for neuroprotective therapy when they become available, although at this time no proven therapies of this kind exist. Patients with idiopathic RBD need to be counseled in regards to this risk and followed for early signs of cerebral neurodegenerative conditions, namely synucleinopathies. This follow-up may include questioning in regards to symptoms; serial neurologic examinations to look for early signs of disease; or more formal testing, such as neuropsychological testing or imaging of the brain.

RBD diagnosis requires not only a clinical history of dream enactment behavior, but also in the sleep laboratory, attended polysomnography demonstrating REM sleep without atonia.[4] In addition to standard chin and lower extremity surface electromyogram recording leads, additional upper extremity electromyogram leads in the arms or shoulders are used to increase sensitivity in identifying REM sleep without atonia.[26] Polysomnography is also useful in ensuring there are no other causes of abnormal movements during sleep, such as periodic limb movements of sleep or sleep-disordered breathing triggering increased muscle tone during REM sleep (pseudo-RBD).

Initial therapy for RBD includes securing the sleep environment and avoiding injury to the patient or bed partner. This includes removing sharp objects and weapons from the bedroom, possibly sleeping in separate beds, moving the bed away from windows, or placing the mattress on the floor. It is also necessary to educate the patient on possible triggers for RBD including medications and sleep deprivation. Treating any underlying primary sleep disorders, such as RLS or sleep-disordered breathing, should also be emphasized. Pharmacologic treatment of RBD includes two major therapies: clonazepam and melatonin.[27] Clonazepam was the first medication shown to be effective in treating RBD. The mechanism of action is unclear. Clonazepam is effective in improving RBD motor activity, but there are significant concerns in older adults in regards to possible side effects of cognitive impairments, sleepiness, and increased risk for falls. Melatonin at high doses has also been shown to improve

RBD symptoms, with less potential for side effects.[28] For refractory cases, combination of melatonin and clonazepam has been used along with a customized bed alarm. Cases series and other small studies demonstrate possible effectiveness of rivastigmine, dopamine agonists, desipramine, clozapine, and carbamazepine.[27]

ALZHEIMER DEMENTIA AND OTHER TAUOPATHIES

Dementia is defined as progressive memory decline and diminished cognition in at least one additional domain: aphasia, apraxia, agnosia, or executive dysfunction. These impairments impact social or occupational functioning. There were an estimated 24 million people in the world with dementia in 2001, with the number expected to double in the next 20 years because of the increase in life expectancy of the population.[29]

Alzheimer disease (AD) is a neurodegenerative condition that causes progressive memory decline and other cognitive deficits. AD is the most common cause of dementia worldwide, and represents approximately 50% to 70% of cases. The neuropathologic hallmark of AD is neuronal loss with cerebral atrophy, β-amyloid plaques, and neurofibrillary tangles composed of tau. There are other neurodegenerative disorders associated with abnormal buildup of tau, including progressive supranuclear palsy (PSP) and corticobasal degeneration. All of these tauopathies are commonly associated with sleep disorders. The same processes that damage areas of the brain causing dementia also cause dysfunction in control of sleep, alertness, and the circadian rhythm. Degeneration of neurons in brain areas, such as nucleus basalis of Meynert, pedunculopontine tegmental and laterodorsal tegmental nuclei, and noradrenergic neurons of the brainstem can lead to reduced REM sleep in AD. Unlike in PD (and other synucleinopathies), RBD is rarely seen in AD.

Degeneration of neurons of the suprachiasmatic nucleus and reduction in melatonin levels in patients with AD has been demonstrated.[30] Further reports suggest that this decrease in melatonin level and disruption of the circadian rhythm may appear early in the course of the disease, and may be potentially responsible for progression of the disease.[31] An interesting association has been reported between sleep disruption or deprivation and β-amyloid levels in normal control subjects, suggesting sleep disruption as an accelerating factor in the progression to AD.[32] One hypothesis is that sleep plays an important role in clearing toxic protein accumulation, such as β-amyloid, in the central nervous system.[33] Sleep changes are also prominent in patients with mild cognitive impairment (MCI), which is a prodromal phase of AD. Studies have shown that up to 60% of patients with MCI have sleep complaints.[34] Patients with MCI were found to have more arousals during slow wave sleep, prolonged REM sleep latency, and increased wake after sleep onset.[35]

Sleep disturbances in AD may also be caused by underlying psychiatric, medical, and primary sleep disturbances; medication-related effects; and insufficient light during the day or excessive light at night before bedtime. Polysomnography studies in patients with AD demonstrate decreased sleep efficiency, percentage slow wave sleep, and REM sleep, and prolonged REM sleep latency.[36] Although some of these may be age-related changes, the findings in AD are more prominent than in age-matched control subjects. Sleep spindles and K-complexes become poorly formed as the condition progresses, making distinction between stage N1 and N2 sleep more difficult in electroencephalography.[37]

Insomnia

Even early in the course of disease, patients with AD complain of disrupted sleep, insomnia, and frequent nighttime awakenings. The insomnia is multifactorial, likely caused by comorbid medical conditions and medication side effects, and damage to areas in the brain that control sleep, wakefulness, and the circadian rhythm. A different hypothesis suggests altered orexin levels in cerebrospinal fluid resulting in sleep dysregulation.[38] Circadian rhythm disorders are seen at higher rates in patients with dementia, because there have been studies demonstrating altered levels of melatonin in these patients and damage to the suprachiasmatic nucleus.[30] Patients generally present clinically with prolonged wakefulness during the night along with excessive sleepiness during the daytime in the forms of naps. This disrupted sleep pattern can cause worsening behavior, confusion, and agitation in the evening and nighttime, which has been called "sundowning." Environmental factors also play a role in exacerbating these symptoms, such as decreased physical exercise and decreased bright light exposure.[39] In patients with dementia in skilled nursing facilities, nocturnal awakenings are exacerbated by roommates, ambient noise, or bed-checks. In addition, exacerbation of any underlying medical issue (ie, infection, metabolic abnormality) can trigger sundowning or worsen sleep. This insomnia and sleep disruption can affect not only the patient, but also the caregiver's sleep and may lead to a visit to an emergency department or placement into a facility if the disruption persists.

Management of insomnia includes educating the patient and caregivers about good sleep hygiene and habits (**Box 3**). Circadian rhythm disorders in patients with AD are treated with properly timed bright light therapy and exogenous melatonin to reset the intrinsic clock to their desired bedtime and wake times. Both nighttime melatonin and morning light exposure for 1 hour improved daytime alertness and reduced sleep disruption in patients with AD.[40] Evidence demonstrates that melatonin at night in this population may improve sleep quality and daytime functioning.[41]

Hypnotics in patients with dementia should be used cautiously. Careful consideration of the benefits versus risks of the pharmacotherapy needs to be assessed. Possible side effects of hypnotics in this age group with dementia include risks of falls and worsened cognition. There are limited studies of hypnotics in patients with dementia, although in practice, many of the same hypnotics used in the general population are used in this specific patient population. These include zolpidem, eszopiclone, zaleplon, ramelteon, and triazolam. Trazodone in low doses is also commonly used and was shown to improve sleep in one small randomized, placebo-controlled study.[42] Melatonin (prolonged release) helped improve sleep in patients with mild to moderate AD in one randomized, placebo-controlled multicenter study.[43]

Obstructive Sleep Apnea

It is unclear if there is a higher incidence of sleep-disordered breathing in patients with AD as compared with age-matched control subjects, although there are numerous studies suggesting a higher risk.[44] The incidence of sleep-disordered breathing in older patients is higher than the general population. There is some evidence to suggest that obstructive sleep apnea may lead to a higher risk or earlier onset of dementia or MCI.[45,46] Diagnosis should be confirmed with objective testing in the form of an in-laboratory attended polysomnography or home sleep apnea test in appropriate patients. Treatment options remain the same as in the general population, including positive airway pressure, weight loss, positional therapy, and oral appliances. CPAP has been shown to reduce subjective daytime sleepiness in AD[47] and decrease arousals and increase stage N3 sleep.[48] CPAP as treatment in patients with AD with sleep apnea has demonstrated improved cognition and slowing of cognitive decline.[49,50] Adherence with CPAP therapy, which is already challenging in the general population, may be even more challenging in patients with dementia given their cognitive deficits and possibly worsening confusion at bedtime.

PROGRESSIVE SUPRANUCLEAR PALSY

Patients suffering from PSP also have numerous sleep complaints. PSP is a neurodegenerative condition caused by abnormal accumulation of tau in the central nervous system. Symptoms include axial rigidity, postural instability, and a supranuclear gaze palsy. Patients with PSP commonly suffer from insomnia for similar reasons as other patients with dementia and neurodegenerative conditions mentioned previously (eg, damage to sleep-controlling areas of the brain, muscle spasms, medication side effects, mood disorder). Sleep studies in patients with PSP have demonstrated reduced REM sleep and spindle formation[51] and frequent arousals.[52] Patients with PSP also have more RLS, which may contribute to insomnia.[53] RBD is noted at high rates in PSP, but not as high as PD or other synucleinopathies.[54]

SUMMARY

Patients suffering from neurodegenerative conditions frequently report sleep complaints, such as insomnia and excessive daytime sleepiness. These symptoms are likely multifactorial, not only caused by their underlying neurologic disorder, but also by medications and other comorbidities associated with the progressive condition. A detailed history, and possibly sleep logs, actigraphy, or polysomnography, may be necessary to properly diagnosis and manage these patients. Improvement in sleep may result in improvement in neurologic symptoms and quality of life in this population. There is growing evidence that disrupted sleep may lead

| Box 3 |
| **Sleep hygiene recommendations** |
| Keep a regular bedtime and wake time throughout the week |
| Engage in relaxing activities (winding down) before bedtime |
| Limit liquids before bedtime |
| Avoid caffeine, tobacco, and alcohol in the evening time |
| Avoid long naps (>30 minutes) during the day |
| Limit exposure to light before bedtime (including light from electronic devices) |
| Make sure sleep environment is quiet and comfortable |

to acceleration in the progression of the neurodegenerative disorder and may play a role in the pathogenesis. RBD may precede the development of clinical symptoms of synucleinopathies, such as PD by years or decades. An awareness of the high prevalence and consequences of sleep disturbance in older adults with neurodegenerative disorders is essential in the management of these important conditions.

REFERENCES

1. de Lau LM, Breteler MM. Epidemiology of Parkinson's disease. Lancet Neurol 2006;5(6):525–35.

2. Tandberg E, Larsen JP, Karlsen K. A community-based study of sleep disorders in patients with Parkinson's disease. Mov Disord 1998;13(6):895–9.

3. Takakusaki K, Saitoh K, Harada H, et al. Evidence for a role of basal ganglia in the regulation of rapid eye movement sleep by electrical and chemical stimulation for the pedunculopontine tegmental nucleus and the substantia nigra pars reticulata in decerebrate cats. Neuroscience 2004;124(1):207–20.

4. American Academy of Seep Medicine. International classification of sleep disorders, 3rd edition: diagnostic and coding manual. Westchester (IL): American Academy of Sleep Medicine; 2014.

5. Pierantozzi M, Placidi F, Liguori C, et al. Rotigotine may improve sleep architecture in Parkinson's disease: a double-blind, randomized, placebo-controlled polysomnographic study. Sleep Med 2016;21:140–4.

6. Ondo W, Vuong K, Jankovic J. Exploring the relationship between Parkinson disease and restless legs syndrome. Arch Neurol 2002;59:421–4.

7. Breen DP, Vuono R, Nawarathna U, et al. Sleep and circadian rhythm regulation in early Parkinson disease. JAMA Neurol 2014;71(5):589–95.

8. Videnovic A, Noble C, Reid KJ, et al. Circadian melatonin rhythm and excessive daytime sleepiness in Parkinson disease. JAMA Neurol 2014; 71(4):463–9.

9. Menza M, Dobkin RD, Marin H, et al. Treatment of insomnia in Parkinson's disease: a controlled trial of eszopiclone and placebo. Mov Disord 2010; 25(11):1708–14.

10. Rios Romenets S, Creti L, Fichten C, et al. Doxepin and cognitive behavioural therapy for insomnia in patients with Parkinson's disease: a randomized study. Parkinsonism Relat Disord 2013;19(7):670–5.

11. Frucht S, Rogers JD, Greene PE, et al. Falling asleep at the wheel: motor vehicle mishaps in persons taking pramipexole and ropinirole. Neurology 1999;52: 1908–10.

12. Abbott RD, Ross GW, White LR, et al. Excessive daytime sleepiness and subsequent development of Parkinson disease. Neurology 2005;65:1442–6.

13. Hobson D, Lang A, Wayne Martin W, et al. Excessive daytime sleepiness and sudden-onset sleep in Parkinson disease. A survey by the Canadian movement disorder group. JAMA 2002; 287:455–63.

14. Arnulf I. Excessive daytime sleepiness and parkinsonism. Sleep Med Rev 2005;9:185–200.

15. Wienecke M, Werth E, Poryazova R, et al. Progressive dopamine and hypocretin deficiencies in Parkinson's disease: is there an impact on sleep and wakefulness? J Sleep Res 2012;21(6):710–7.

16. Postuma RB, Lang AE, Munhoz RP, et al. Caffeine for treatment of Parkinson disease: a randomized controlled trial. Neurology 2012;79:651–8.

17. Ondo WG, Fayle R, Atassi F, et al. Modafinil for daytime somnolence in Parkinson's disease: double blind, placebo controlled parallel trial. J Neurol Neurosurg Psychiatry 2005;76:1636–9.

18. Ondo WG, Perkins T, Swick T, et al. Sodium oxybate for excessive daytime sleepiness in Parkinson disease: an open-label polysomnographic study. Arch Neurol 2008;65(10):1337–40.

19. Trotti LM, Bliwise DL. No increased risk of obstructive sleep apnea in Parkinson's disease. Mov Disord 2010;25(13):2246–9.

20. Neikrug AB, Liu L, Avanzino JA, et al. Continuous positive airway pressure improves sleep and daytime sleepiness in patients with Parkinson disease and sleep apnea. Sleep 2014;37(1):177–85.

21. Shimohata T, Nakayama H, Aizawa N, et al. Discontinuation of continuous positive airway pressure treatment in multiple system atrophy. Sleep Med 2014;15(9):1147–9.

22. Silber MH, Levine S. Stridor and death in multiple system atrophy. Mov Disord 2000;15(4):699–704.

23. Palma JA, Fernandez-Cordon C, Coon EA, et al. Prevalence of REM sleep behavior disorder in multiple system atrophy: a multicenter study and meta-analysis. Clin Auton Res 2015;25(1):69–75.

24. Sixel-Doring F, Trautmann F, Mollenhauer B, et al. Associated factors for REM sleep behavior disorder in Parkinson disease. Neurology 2011;77:1048–54.

25. Iranzo A, Fernandez-Arcos A, Tolosa E, et al. Neurodegenerative disorder risk in idiopathic REM sleep behavior disorder: study in 174 patients. PLoS One 2014;9:e89741.

26. Frauscher B, Iranzo A, Hogl B, et al. Quantification of electromyographic activity during REM sleep in multiple muscles in REM sleep behavior disorder. Sleep 2008;31:724–31.

27. Aurora RN, Zak RS, Maganti RK, et al. Best practice guide for the treatment of REM sleep behavior disorder (RBD). J Clin Sleep Med 2010;6:85–95.

28. Kunz D, Mahlberg R. A two-part, double-blind, placebo-controlled trial of exogenous melatonin in REM sleep behaviour disorder. J Sleep Res 2010; 19:591–6.

29. Plassman BL, Langa KM, Fisher GG, et al. Preva-
    lence of dementia in the United States: the aging,
    demographics, and memory study. Neuroepidemiol-
    ogy 2007;29(1–2):125–32.

30. Mishima K, Tozawa T, Satoh K, et al. Melatonin
    secretion rhythm disorders in patients with senile de-
    mentia of Alzheimer's type with disturbed sleep-
    waking. Biol Psychiatry 1999;45(4):417–21.

31. Bedrosian TA, Nelson RJ. Pro: Alzheimer's disease
    and circadian dysfunction: chicken or egg? Alz-
    heimers Res Ther 2012;4(4):25.

32. Spira AP, Gamaldo AA, An Y, et al. Self-reported
    sleep and beta-amyloid deposition in community-
    dwelling older adults. JAMA Neurol 2013;70(12):
    1537–43.

33. Xie L, Kang H, Xu Q, et al. Sleep drives metabolite
    clearance from the adult brain. Science 2013;342:
    373–7.

34. Beaulieu-Bonneau S, Hudon C. Sleep disturbances
    in older adults with mild cognitive impairment. Int
    Psychogeriatr 2009;21:654–66.

35. Westerberg CE, Mander BA, Florczak SM, et al.
    Concurrent impairments in sleep and memory in am-
    nestic mild cognitive impairment. J Int Neuropsychol
    Soc 2012;18:490–500.

36. Bliwise DL. Sleep in normal aging and dementia.
    Sleep 1993;16(1):40–81.

37. Ktonas PY, Golemati S, Xanthopoulos P, et al. Poten-
    tial dementia biomarkers based on the time-varying
    microstructure of sleep EEG spindles. Conf Proc
    IEEE Eng Med Biol Soc 2007;2007:2464–7.

38. Liquori C, Romigi A, Nuccetelli M, et al. Orexinergic
    system dysregulation, sleep impairment, and cogni-
    tive decline in Alzheimer disease. JAMA Neurol
    2014;71(12):1498–505.

39. Sullivan SC, Richards KC. Predictors of circadian
    sleep-wake rhythm maintenance in elders with de-
    mentia. Aging Ment Health 2004;8(2):143–52.

40. Dowling GA, Burr RL, Van Someren EJ, et al. Mela-
    tonin and bright-light treatment for rest-activity
    disruption in institutionalized patients with Alz-
    heimer's disease. J Am Geriatr Soc 2008;56(2):
    239–46.

41. de Jonghe A, Korevaar JC, van Munster BC, et al.
    Effectiveness of melatonin treatment on circadian
    rhythm disturbances in dementia. Are there implica-
    tions for delirium? A systematic review. Int J Geriatr
    Psychiatry 2010;25(12):1201–8.

42. Camargos EF, Louzada LL, Quintas JL, et al. Traza-
    done improves sleep parameters in Alzheimer

    disease patients: a randomized, double-blind, and
    placebo controlled study. Am J Geriatr Psychiatry
    2014;22(12):1565–74.

43. Wade AG, Farmer M, Harari G, et al. Add-on pro-
    longed release melatonin for cognitive function and
    sleep in mild to moderate Alzheimer's disease: a 6
    month randomized, placebo-controlled, multicenter
    trial. Clin Interv Aging 2014;9:947–61.

44. Ancoli-Israel S, Klauber MR, Butters N, et al. Demen-
    tia in institutionalized elderly: relation to sleep ap-
    nea. J Am Geriatr Soc 1991;39(3):258–63.

45. Yaffe K, Laffan AM, Harrison SL, et al. Sleep-disor-
    dered breathing, hypoxia, and risk of mild cognitive
    impairment and dementia in older women. JAMA
    2011;306(6):613–9.

46. Osorio RS, Gumb T, Pirraglia E, et al. Sleep-disor-
    dered breathing advances cognitive decline in the
    elderly. Neurology 2015;84(19):1964–71.

47. Chong MS, Ayalon L, Marler M, et al. Continuous
    positive airway pressure reduces subjective daytime
    sleepiness in patients with mild to moderate Alz-
    heimer's disease with sleep disordered breathing.
    J Am Geriatr Soc 2006;54(5):777–81.

48. Cooke JR, Ancoli-Israel S, Liu L, et al. Continuous
    positive airway pressure deepens sleep in patients
    with Alzheimer's disease and obstructive sleep ap-
    nea. Sleep Med 2009;10(10):1101–6.

49. Troussiere AC, Monaca CC, Salleron J, et al. Treat-
    ment of sleep apnea syndrome decreases cognitive
    decline in patients with Alzheimer's disease.
    J Neurol Neurosurg Psychiatry 2014;85(12):1405–8.

50. Ancoli-Israel S, Palmer BW, Cooke JR, et al. Cogni-
    tive effects of treating obstructive sleep apnea in
    Alzheimer's disease: a randomized controlled study.
    J Am Geriatr Soc 2008;56(11):2076–81.

51. Petit D, Gagnon JF, Fantini ML, et al. Sleep and
    quantitative EEG in neurodegenerative disorders.
    J Psychosom Res 2004;56(5):487–96.

52. Aldrich MS, Foster NL, White RF, et al. Sleep abnor-
    malities in progressive supranuclear palsy. Ann Neu-
    rol 1989;25(6):577–81.

53. Gama RL, Tavora DG, Bomfim RC, et al. Sleep dis-
    turbances and brain MRI morphometry in Parkin-
    son's disease, multiple system atrophy and
    progressive supranuclear palsy: a comparative
    study. Parkinsonism Relat Disord 2010;16:275–9.

54. Sixel-Doring F, Schweitzer M, Mollenhauer B, et al.
    Polysomnographic findings, video-based sleep
    analysis and sleep perception in progressive supra-
    nuclear palsy. Sleep Med 2009;10(4):407–15.

Chronic Medical Conditions and Sleep in the Older Adult

Saban-Hakki Onen, MD, PhD[a,b,*], Fannie Onen, MD, PhD[c,d]

KEYWORDS

- Sleep disturbance • Sleep apnea • Chronic disease • Medical condition • Falls • Pain • Cancer
- Heart failure

KEY POINTS

- The older population with chronic medical conditions and sleep disturbances is clinically heterogeneous and complex, making the management of sleep disturbances challenging.
- Pain and medications to treat pain can disturb sleep. Sleep disturbances may adversely affect the course of chronic painful diseases in adults of advanced age.
- Cancer-related pain, fears, anxiety and depression, and cancer therapy are correlated with sleep complaints in older patients with cancer. Sleep disturbance may negatively affect cancer.
- Falls are prevalent in the older population with insomnia and those with sleep apnea; sedative hypnotics increase the risk of falls. Treating sleep disorders may help prevent falls.
- Chronic heart failure may contribute to sleep apnea and sleep apnea may impair cardiac function chronically.

INTRODUCTION

Demographic changes in the United States, Europe, and Asia are leading to an aging population with disability and chronic medical conditions. For example, 3 of 4 Americans aged 65 and over have at least 2 concurrent chronic conditions.[1] Chronic condition is a general term that includes chronic illnesses and impairments that last a year or more and require ongoing medical attention and/or limit activities of daily living.[2] A wide range of chronic medical conditions can have an impact on the structure and distribution of sleep in the older adult. However, in some cases sleep disturbance and its treatment may also trigger or worsen medical conditions. Sleep disturbance has been reported in as many as 40% to 50% of older Americans aged 65 years and over.[3] Sleep problems associated with other chronic medical conditions may have strong adverse effects on health status, function, and quality of life; and may require complex health care management, decision making, and/or coordination. Overall, the older population with chronic medical conditions and sleep disturbance is characterized by tremendous clinical heterogeneity and complexity (ie, number, severity, and type of medical conditions, and their treatments). Thus, the management of sleep disturbance in late life is challenging. This article reviews frequently encountered medical conditions in everyday practice and examines the consequences of these

Disclosure Statement: The authors have nothing to disclose.
[a] Geriatric Sleep Medicine Center, Eduard Herriot University Hospital, HCL, Lyon 69003, France; [b] INSERM 1028, University of Lyon, Lyon, France; [c] Department of Geriatrics, Bichat University Hospital, APHP, Paris 75018, France; [d] INSERM 1178 and CESP, University of Paris-Sud, Paris, France
* Corresponding author. Geriatric Sleep Medicine Center, Eduard Herriot University Hospital, HCL, Lyon 69003, France.
E-mail address: saban-hakki.onen@chu-lyon.fr

sleep.theclinics.com

conditions on sleep in the older adult, and reviews the possible impact of sleep disturbance on these common medical conditions. Finally, strategies to improve sleep disturbance in older patients with comorbid medical conditions are formulated according to available data and our clinical experiences. These frequently encountered medical conditions include, but are not limited to, pain, falls, cancer, and congestive heart failure (CHF).

CHRONIC MEDICAL CONDITIONS AND SLEEP INTERACTIONS
Pain

Clinical aspects and dual relationship between pain and sleep disturbance

Pain is probably the most frequent and disabling symptom in medicine. It is an unpleasant sensory and emotional experience, and has close connections with consciousness or awareness as well as sleep.[4,5] Most cross-sectional epidemiologic studies have shown that the overall prevalence of pain increases with advancing age. In late life, pain is a very common problem, affecting more than 50% of older persons living in the community, and more than 80% of nursing home residents.[6,7] In the older population, pain is commonly a symptom of 1 or more existing health conditions. Cross-sectional research in clinical samples, as well as experimental studies in healthy adults, suggest that the relationship between pain and sleep are robust and bidirectionally connected under the influence of cognitive and neurobiological changes.[8–10]

The impact of pain on sleep and sleep disturbance is widely studied. Almost any painful illness, both in middle-aged[11–13] and older adults,[14] has been associated with sleep disturbance. Insomnia characterized by a difficulty in initiating or maintaining sleep is often associated with pain. Thus, among 50 community-dwelling older adults with insomnia (mean age, 69 years), Dzierzewski and colleagues[10] found that objectively measured nocturnal sleep and subjective report of morning pain show day-to-day associations and covary over time. In addition, a cross-sectional epidemiologic survey by means of questionnaires was conducted in 430 older Icelanders aged 65 and over.[15] The authors reported a significant relationship between difficulty initiating sleep, difficulty maintaining sleep and early morning awakening, and being awakened by pain. There was, however, no significant effect of pain on total sleep time. In another cross-sectional survey from Australia, insomnia was associated with frequent pain and poor physical health among 874 community-dwelling and 59 institutional residents aged 70 years and over.[16]

Several cross-sectional studies have investigated the relationship between self-reported sleep disturbances and pain related to osteoarthritis (OA). OA is a common health condition affecting mainly older adults that causes chronic joint pain and sleep disturbance with deterioration of quality of life.[9] OA-related pain is the most common factor predicting sleep disturbance in up to 60% of patients.[17] Usually, this pain tends to be exacerbated in the evening and on awakening, and lasts 20 to 30 minutes. Among persons with knee OA, up to 31% report significant disturbances in initiating sleep and 81% have difficulties maintaining nighttime sleep.[8,18] In the same way, lumbar spine and hip OA with pain have also been reported to delay sleep onset and impair sleep maintenance. The findings of sleep fragmentation owing to an increased number of arousals[19] and periodic limb movements[20] may in part explain the fatigue and joint stiffness experienced upon awakening, which are frequently reported by these patients. One-year longitudinal relationships of sleep difficulties with pain, depression, and functional disability have been studied in 288 older adults (mean age at inclusion 67.9 years) with physician-diagnosed knee OA. Longitudinal analyses used baseline sleep disturbance to predict the 1-year change in pain, disability, and depression.[21] Cross-sectional analyses revealed a significant association of sleep disturbance with pain and depression, but not functional disability. The sleep–pain relationship was wholly explained by depressive symptoms; in contrast, depression was significantly and independently associated with both pain and sleep problems. Furthermore, sleep disturbance exacerbated effects of pain on depression, such that depressive symptoms were greatest among those with both significant sleep problems and higher than average pain. In 1-year longitudinal analyses, sleep problems predicted increases in depression and disability, but not pain.

Clinical investigations concerning the impact of sleep disturbance on pain perception and tolerance and painful illness are scarce. If patients with acute or chronic painful conditions often suffer from sleep disturbances, changes in sleep pattern could also influence pain tolerance.[22] Sleep is an important homeostatic feature and, when impaired, contributes to the development or worsening of painful conditions. According to experimental studies in both animals and humans, sleep deprivation produces hyperalgesic changes.[23] Furthermore, sleep rebound consecutive to experimental sleep deprivation induces an increase in the pain threshold (analgesic effect) in healthy volunteers and animals.[23] The relationship between obstructive sleep apnea (OSA), which is a chronic sleep deprivation model, and pain tolerance has been studied by our team in adults aged 70 years and older. In this randomized, double-blind crossover study, when older sleep apnea patients have been treated with continuous positive airway pressure (CPAP), the tolerance to electrical pain was significantly improved.[24] We speculated that, among chronically sleep-deprived older OSA patients, CPAP treatment possibly induced more restorative slow wave sleep with less sleep fragmentation (ie, less arousal). Because CPAP therapy improves respiratory parameters during sleep, another plausible mechanism may be that appropriate nocturnal oxygenation might increase pain thresholds (ie, an analgesic effect) in older OSA patients. In a case control study (158 older vs 1166 middle-aged adults), Tarasiuk and colleagues[25] aimed to determine whether older subjects with OSA had different morbidity and health care use than both older subjects without OSA and middle-aged patients with OSA. Using a multiple logistic regression analysis (adjusting for age, body mass index, and apnea–hypopnea index), the authors demonstrated that older patients aged 67 and over with untreated OSA (apnea–hypopnea index >5 per hour, reduced total sleep time, reduced sleep efficiency) have high health care use and increased pain medication consumption compared with all other groups.

Interventions to improve comorbid sleep disturbance and pain

Many factors, including pain, the painful disease process, and medications, can disturb sleep, and sleep disturbances may also adversely affect the natural course of the painful disease in older adults. Improving sleep quantity and quality in patients with painful disorders may break this vicious circle and, as a consequence, enhance the patients' overall health and quality of life. When formulating a treatment plan, one needs to be aware of the important influence of concurrent medications (eg, hypnotics and sedating pain medications) and the potential impact of comorbid medical (eg, sleep apnea) and cognitive problems.

Alleviating pain may improve sleep; however, certain analgesics, such as opioids, can disturb sleep. Sleep disturbances secondary to chronic opioid drug use and abuse have been described in small samples of patients with substance abuse problems and middle-aged adults. Opioids are known to reduce sleep time, decrease sleep efficiency, increase sleep latency, increase sleep fragmentation, and reduce restorative slow wave

sleep.[26] As a vicious cycle, opioid-related sleep impairment may increase pain and create a need for more analgesics. It is important to manage pain in older patients with sleep apnea cautiously. They are exquisitely sensitive to muscle relaxants and central nervous system depressant drugs, with upper airway obstruction or respiratory arrest occurring even using minimal doses. Benzodiazepines and opioids should be avoided, especially if patients are not treated with CPAP devices.

Older patients with significant pain who may be candidates for opioid or benzodiazepine therapy should be screened for sleep apnea, with questionnaires such as the Observation-based Nocturnal Sleep Inventory.[27] It is recommended that patients with a positive Observation-based Nocturnal Sleep Inventory (ie, at least 2 episodes of snoring or at least 1 episode of apnea observed during the 5 night-time standardized visits) should undergo overnight sleep testing for sleep apnea. For patients with positive Observation-based Nocturnal Sleep Inventory who have not been tested (or treated) for sleep apnea, it is appropriate to analyze the risks and benefits of sedative drug therapy and in some cases avoid opioid analgesics or benzodiazepines during the night time period. Although many antidepressants, including serotonin reuptake inhibitors and serotonin–norepinephrine reuptake inhibitors also degrade sleep architecture and worsen restless legs syndrome, psychiatric symptoms may still justify the use of these medications.

For mild to moderate sleep disturbance with pain, sleep hygiene and cognitive–behavioral therapy may be an alternative to pharmacotherapy. Cognitive–behavioral therapy for insomnia improved both immediate and long-term self-reported sleep and pain in a sample of 23 older patients (mean age of 69 years) with comorbid insomnia and OA.[28] These results suggest that nonpharmacologic improvement of sleep, per se, in patients with OA may result in decreased pain.

Cancer

Clinical aspects and dual relationship between cancer and sleep disturbance

Advanced age is a significant risk factor for cancer, with persons over 65 years accounting for 60% of newly diagnosed malignancies and 70% of all cancer deaths.[29,30] Sleep complaints including insomnia, poor sleep quality, and short sleep duration are prominent concerns of patients with cancer. Although the prevalence of sleep disturbance varies among studies because of the heterogeneity of populations studied, between one-third and one-half of newly diagnosed patients with cancer experience sleep problems.[31] In a large cross-sectional survey, patients with various cancers (mean age, 65 years) reported leg restlessness (41%), insomnia (31%), and excessiveness daytime sleepiness (28%).[32] These subjective complaints are correlated with objective sleep recordings and patients with cancer are frequently found to have increased sleep latency (difficulty falling asleep), fragmented sleep, reduced total sleep time, and low sleep efficiency (the ratio of time asleep over total time in bed).[33] The etiology of sleep disturbance in patients with cancer is typically multifactorial in nature.[34] Older people with cancer may already have sleep problems owing to poor sleep hygiene or lifestyle issues, or may already be diagnosed with a common sleep disorder such as sleep apnea or restless legs syndrome. In addition, cancer-related pain, cancer-related fears, anxiety and depression, previous non–cancer-related comorbid conditions, the type and stage of the cancer, and treatment side effects such as nausea, vomiting, or diarrhea are common factors precipitating or worsening sleep problems.[31,35] Conversely, sleep disturbance may negatively affect cancer by increasing fatigue, pain, and discomfort, and reducing emotional well-being.[35]

Interventions to improve sleep disturbance for patients with cancer

According to a phone survey conducted among 150 patients at various stages of treatment for breast and lung cancer, 44% of them experienced sleep disturbances on most nights in the past month and they reported that health care providers typically never asked about their sleep.[36] In other large surveys of psychotropic drug consumption among oncology patients, rates of hypnotic prescriptions were around 43% to 48%,[37,38] and 25% of patients have received drugs for nausea and vomiting.[38] Many health care providers are concerned about overall well-being of their older patients, and prescribe in some cases a hypnotic for potential sleep problems precipitated by anxiety, depression, or painful investigations at the time of initial cancer diagnosis. Because hypnotics may be less effective after a few weeks of continued use, patients should be informed that the prescription is indicated for short-term use, and will probably be most helpful during the peak period of treatment or during painful procedures.[34] In older patients with cancer with persistent sleep complaints, sedative antidepressants and anxiolytics introduced at bed time may be an alternative to hypnotics. In addition, because of the poor prognosis in late stage cancer, short-acting hypnotics

including benzodiazepines and adequate pain management even with opioids may be more effective for the management of sleep problems.

Falls

Clinical aspects and relationship between falls, insomnia, sedative drugs, and sleep apnea

Falls and fall-related injuries in older people are a leading cause of mortality, morbidity, and premature nursing home placement.[39,40] It is estimated that falls occur yearly in one-third of persons over the age of 65[39] and represent a significant economic burden.[40,41] Several studies have reported an association between nocturnal sleep disturbance, daytime sleepiness, inadequate use of medications, and risk of falls.

In the Study of Osteoporotic Fractures (SOF) involving 8101 community-dwelling older women, Stone and colleagues[42] found that self-reported long sleep and daily napping were associated with greater risk of falls and fractures even after accounting for a variety of potential confounding or explanatory variables such as age, body mass index, medication use, comorbidities, urinary incontinence, cognitive function, depression, and lifestyle factors. The association between daily napping and risk of falls was independent of antidepressant use, lower extremity strength, and nighttime sleep quality. A German phone survey of 4127 community-dwelling older adults have confirmed previous findings that sleep disturbances might be related to falls in the older population.[43] The associations between trouble falling asleep, trouble staying asleep, and a trend toward longer sleep duration and falls are most frequently present in subgroups, especially in participants aged 76 years and older and in individuals without dizziness. Other data analyses from participants in the Osteoporotic Fractures in Men Study[44] found that subjective and objective sleep disturbances were associated with an increased risk of incident falls in a sample of 3101 community-dwelling older men. When considering actigraphic short sleep duration, sleep efficiency, daytime sleepiness, and nocturnal hypoxemia together, daytime sleepiness and nocturnal hypoxemia (but not apnea–hypopnea index) were independently associated with recurrent falls. A metaanalysis of the impact of different medication classes on falls in older people was performed.[44] More than 79,000 participants were located in long-term care facilities, hospital acute medical facilities, or in the community. The mean age ranged from 65 to 90 years. The authors of this review concluded that the use of sedatives and hypnotics, antidepressants, and benzodiazepines showed a significant association with falls in older people. Another metaanalysis involving 2417 participants aged 60 or over has found that, among patients complaining of insomnia, improvements in sleep with sedative use are statistically significant, but the magnitude of the effect is small.[45] The increased risk of adverse events is statistically significant and potentially clinically relevant in older people at risk of falls and cognitive impairment. Despite the negative impact of sedative drugs on falls in previous studies, in an observational study of 34,163 nursing home residents (mean age 84 years) in Michigan, Avidan and colleagues[46] have found that untreated insomnia or hypnotic-treated unresponsive insomnia also predicts falls. Similarly, a survey of 150 Australian nursing home residents (mean age, 82 years) found that poor self-reported sleep quality and nocturnal awakenings, but not the use of hypnotics, were associated with an increased risk of falls.[47] The effects of 26-hour experimental sleep deprivation (experimental insomnia) on postural control and their modulation by attentional resources and visual input in 15 young (age range, 20–28 years) and 15 older adults (age range 60–70 years) have been studied.[48] It was concluded that sleep loss has greater destabilizing effects on postural control in older than in younger participants, and may therefore increase the risk of falls in older people. In sleep-deprived older adults, postural instability was more pronounced under poor visual conditions. Finally, in a case series from our team, 4 older patients with recurrent falls, OSA, excessive daytime sleepiness, and CPAP treatment were followed for 2 years.[49] A causal relationship was found between OSA and injury related to falling asleep in these older patients. Treatment of OSA with CPAP improved attention, daytime vigilance, and consequently gait and balance control and prevented falls in all these patients.

Taken together, these results suggest that there may be multiple pathways by which disturbed sleep may increase risk of falls. In older adults with sleep disturbance, fall mechanisms are likely to be multifactorial, including impaired balance and/or reaction time arising from insufficient sleep, sleep apnea–related hypoxemia and sleep fragmentation with consequent daytime sleepiness, increased postural instability during dark hours, and the residual daytime effects of medications used to treat sleep problems. This leads to a situation where both insomnia itself and the medications used to treat it, as well as sleep apnea, may all contribute to the increased risk of falls.

Interventions to improve sleep disturbance in older fallers

Insomnia, daytime sleepiness, sleep apnea with nocturnal hypoxemia, and drug treatments for insomnia have been associated with increased risk of falls in the older population, both in the institutional setting and in community-dwelling populations. Appropriate treatment of insomnia in older adults may help prevent falls. However, the increased risk of falls owing to overuse of sedative drugs, especially benzodiazepines and benzodiazepine-like medications (eg, zolpidem, zopiclone, and zaleplon) should always be considered when treating insomnia in older patient populations. In older people, the benefits of these drugs may not justify the increased risk, particularly if the patient has additional risk factors for cognitive or psychomotor adverse events. In addition, treating older recurrent fallers with sleep apnea may alleviate their nocturnal hypoxemia and reduce excessive daytime sleepiness and prevent falls. Thus, recurrent fallers should be screened for sleep apnea.[27]

Chronic Heart Failure

Clinical aspects and dual relationship between congestive heart failure and sleep disturbance

The lifetime risk of developing CHF is around 20%[50] and its prevalence and incidence increase with age, particularly in individuals older than 80 years.[51] CHF is the final common stage of many diseases of the heart. It is exacerbated by neurohormonal imbalance and punctuated by acute episodes leading to repetitive hospitalizations and poor outcomes for older patients. Some patients have CHF owing to left ventricular systolic dysfunction which is associated with reduced left ventricular ejection fraction (EF); this is termed heart failure with reduced EF (HFrEF). Others have heart failure with preserved EF (HFpEF) and demonstrable diastolic abnormalities.

In addition to increased CHF in older adults, sleep-related breathing disorders, including central sleep apnea (CSA) and OSA also are known to increase with advancing age. For ages 70 to 99 years, the prevalence of sleep-related breathing disorders defined as an apnea–hypopnea index of 15 or greater per hour of sleep is about 20%.[52] Several epidemiologic studies focusing mainly on HFrEF suggest that both CSA and OSA are common in the CHF population. However, the prevalence of sleep apnea in CHF varies according to the apnea–hypopnea index threshold applied in each study. In a US-based prospective study of 81 ambulatory male patients with stable HFrEF, the prevalence of sleep apnea defined by an apnea–hypopnea index of 20 or more events per hour was 51% (40% CSA and 11% OSA).[53] Patients with sleep apnea have a high prevalence of atrial fibrillation and ventricular arrhythmias. Later, a large retrospective sleep study in 450 consecutive patients with HFrEF from Canada reported a 61% prevalence of sleep apnea using criteria of 15 events per hour or greater. The prevalence of OSA was higher in this study (32%) than that of CSA (29%), likely owing to selection bias (suspicion of OSA was 1 criterion for referral to the sleep laboratory) or owing to the retrospective nature of the study.[54] A prospective sleep study from Italy demonstrated a 55% prevalence of CSA with Cheyne–Stokes respiration pattern in 62 patients with HFrEF.[55] Screening for sleep apnea was performed in 700 patients with symptomatic CHF receiving therapy according to current heart failure guidelines (eg, widespread use of β-blockers) involving cardiorespiratory polygraphy.[56] Sleep apnea was present in 76% of patients (40% CSA, 36% OSA). CSA patients were more symptomatic and had a lower EF than OSA patients. Data on sleep-disordered breathing in patients with HFpEF are scarce. In a prospective study evaluating a stable population of patients with CHF selected from a Norwegian heart failure clinic, patients with HFpEF had nearly the same high prevalence of sleep apnea as the group with HFrEF (80% vs 82%).[57] Unlike the patients with HFrEF, the predominant type of sleep-disordered breathing in patients with HFpEF was OSA (62%). Subjects with HFpEF and OSA had a higher body mass index and more likely hypertension compared with patients with HFpEF without OSA. Another prospective study from Germany evaluated 244 consecutive patients with HFpEF and found the overall prevalence of sleep apnea was 70%, with approximately 40% OSA and 30% CSA. Similar to HFrEF, CSA was associated with more severe heart failure.[58] This paper established that the prevalence of sleep apnea in patients with HFpEF is probably as high as HFrEF patients. Whether sleep apnea is of prognostic relevance in HFpEF needs to be determined.

Various lines of evidence suggest that CHF may contribute to sleep-disordered breathing by different mechanisms, including increased pharyngeal wall edema reinforced by nocturnal fluid displacement from the legs to the neck, and unstable ventilatory control. Yumino and colleagues[59] suggest that nocturnal rostral fluid shift contributes to the pathogenesis of both OSA and CSA in patients with CHF. Among their 57 patients with heart failure (EF ≤45%), the magnitude of overnight rostral fluid movement contributed to the severity of 2 types of sleep apnea. This fluid shift was directly related to the degree of leg edema and sitting time and inversely related to the degree of physical activity. Thus, sedentary living may contribute to the pathogenesis of sleep apnea in heart failure not only by facilitating weight gain, but by promoting dependent fluid retention. Patients with CSA (Cheyne-Stokes respiration) in CHF have, in general, a chronic respiratory alkalosis owing to hyperventilation both during wakefulness and sleep. The key pathophysiologic mechanism triggering Cheyne-Stokes respiration is hyperventilation and hypocapnia (low $Paco_2$) that, when below the apneic threshold, triggers a central apnea.[60] Sleep apnea may also impair cardiac function acutely by increasing afterload, caused by an increased ventricular transmural pressure during ongoing negative intrathoracic pressure swings (respiratory efforts); and chronically by increasing sympathetic activity and oxidative stress related to fluctuations in arterial oxygen and carbon dioxide levels and recurrent awakenings, leading to increased blood pressure, nocturnal arrhythmias, and stroke.[61]

Interventions to improve sleep apnea (central and obstructive sleep apnea) for patients with congestive heart failure

For patients with CHF, there is a paucity of data from prospective, randomized, controlled trials addressing the potential benefits of treatment for either OSA or CSA. As such, there are no consensus guidelines endorsed by either sleep medicine or heart failure specialists on management strategies for sleep-disordered breathing associated with CHF.[62] However, the first step in the management plan for a patient with sleep-disordered breathing and CHF should be optimization of CHF treatment using diuretics and beta-blockers. General measures such as avoiding supine sleeping position, reduction of pharyngeal edema (fluid shift), and avoidance of the use of benzodiazepines and other sedatives before bedtime may decrease the likelihood of upper airway occlusion during sleep, thus reducing OSA in patients with CHF. Despite these alternative therapies and the absence of consensus, many patients with CHF will require CPAP to eliminate obstructive and central apneas. Adaptive servoventilation (a therapy that uses a noninvasive ventilator to treat CSA by delivering servocontrolled inspiratory pressure support on top of expiratory positive airway pressure) was proposed as an alternative to CPAP to treat CSA. However, results from the Adaptive Servo-Ventilation for Central Sleep Apnea in Systolic Heart Failure (SERVE-HF) study, reported recently,[63] found that adaptive servoventilation had no significant effect on the primary endpoint in patients who had HFrEF and predominantly CSA, but all-cause and cardiovascular mortality were both increased with this therapy. Owing to detrimental effects of this particular type of positive airway pressure delivery, and the recommendations of all major pulmonary and sleep societies to abstain from servoventilation treatment in patients with HFrEF (EF ≤45%), no recommendation can be given regarding positive airway pressure treatment for this patient group until further trials are available to address mortality effects of PAP in this population.[64]

SUMMARY

Older adults with chronic medical conditions frequently report difficulty initiating sleep, difficulty maintaining sleep, daytime sleepiness, and fatigue. Many chronic medical conditions and medications used to treat these conditions may disturb sleep, and sleep disturbance and its specific treatment (eg, hypnotics) may also adversely affect the natural course of many chronic medical conditions in adults of advanced age. Older adults with sleep disturbance and comorbid medical conditions have an increased risk of mortality, increased risk of hospitalization, and may also receive inappropriate polypharmacy. Existing sleep disorder management strategies in older adults are often limited by a disease-specific focus (eg, insomnia, OSA, periodic limb movement). Sleep disturbance and chronic disease states must be managed concurrently to optimize improvement in quality of life and functioning. In addition to sleep history, evaluation of the older patient's medical history, psychiatric history, and lifestyle and environmental factors should be considered carefully when considering treatment modalities. Management approaches should account for patient and family preferences, and consider prognosis and interactions within and among treatments and conditions.

REFERENCES

1. Gerteis J, Izrael D, Deitz D, et al. Multiple chronic conditions chartbook. AHRQ Publications No, Q14-0038. Rockville (MD): Agency for Healthcare Research and Quality; 2014.
2. Warshaw G. Introduction: advances and challenges in care of older people with chronic illness. Generation 2006;30:5–10.
3. Foley DJ, Monjan AA, Brown SL, et al. Sleep complaints among elderly persons: an epidemiologic study of three communities. Sleep 1995;18:425–32.
4. Bromm B. Consciousness, pain and cortical activity. In: Bromm B, Desmedt JE, editors. Pain and brain:

5. Onen SH. Douleur. In: Onen SH, Onen F, editors. Dictionnaire de médecine du sommeil. Paris: Ellipses; 1998. p. 74 [Context Link].
6. Ferrell BA, Ferrell BR, Rivera L. Pain in cognitively impaired nursing home patients. J Pain Symptom Manage 1995;10:591–8.
7. Helme RD, Gibson SJ. The epidemiology of pain in elderly people. Clin Geriatr Med 2001;17:417–31.
8. Wilcox S, Brenes GA, Levine D, et al. Factors related to sleep disturbance in older adults experiencing knee pain or knee pain with radiographic evidence of knee osteoarthritis. J Am Geriatr Soc 2000;48:1241–51.
9. Smith MT, Quartana PJ, Okonkwo RM, et al. Mechanisms by which sleep disturbance contributes to osteoarthritis pain: a conceptual model. Curr Pain Headache Rep 2009;13:447–54.
10. Dzierzewski JM, Williams JM, Roditi D, et al. Daily variations in objective nighttime sleep and subjective morning pain in older adults with insomnia: evidence of covariation over time. J Am Geriatr Soc 2010;58:925–30.
11. McCracken LM, Iverson GL. Disrupted sleep patterns and daily functioning in patients with chronic pain. Pain Res Manag 2002;7(2):75–9.
12. Moldofsky H. Sleep and pain. Sleep Med Rev 2001;5(5):385–96.
13. Lavigne GL, McMillan D, Zucconi M. Pain and sleep. In: Kryger MH, Roth T, Dement WC, editors. Principles and practice of sleep medicine. 4th edition. Philadelphia: Elsevier Saunders; 2005. p. 1246–55.
14. Mallon L, Hetta J. A survey of sleep habits and sleeping difficulties in an elderly Swedish population. Ups J Med Sci 1997;102:185–97.
15. Gíslason T, Reynisdóttir H, Kristbjarnarson H, et al. Sleep habits and sleep disturbances among the elderly–an epidemiological survey. J Intern Med 1993;234:31–9.
16. Henderson S, Jorm AF, Scott LR, et al. Insomnia in the elderly: its prevalence and correlates in the general population. Med J Aust 1995;162:22–4.
17. Foley D, Ancoli-Israel S, Britz P, et al. Sleep disturbance and chronic disease in older adults: results of the 2003 National Sleep Foundation Sleep in America Survey. J Psychosom Res 2004;56:497–502.
18. Allen KD, Renner JB, Devellis B, et al. Osteoarthritis and sleep: the Johnston County osteoarthritis project. J Rheumatol 2008;35:1102–7.
19. Parmelee PA. Assessment of pain in the elderly. In: Lawton MP, Teresi J, editors. Annual review of gerontology and geriatrics. New York: Springer; 1994. p. 281–301.
20. Meenan RF, Mason JH, Anderson JJ, et al. AIMS2. The content and properties of a revised and

from nociception to cognition. New York: Raven Press; 1995. p. 35–59 [Context Link].

expanded arthritis impact measurement scales health status questionnaire. Arthritis Rheum 1992; 35:1–10.

21. Parmelee PA, Tighe Caitlan A. Dautovich ND. Sleep disturbance in osteoarthritis: linkages with pain, disability, and depressive symptoms. Arthritis Care Res (Hoboken) 2015;67:358–65.

22. Onen SH, Alloui A, Gross A, et al. The effects of total sleep deprivation, selective sleep interruption and sleep recovery on pain tolerance thresholds in healthy subjects. J Sleep Res 2001;10:35–42.

23. Lautenbacher S, Kundermann B, Krieg JC. Sleep deprivation and pain perception. Sleep Med Rev 2006;10:357–69.

24. Onen SH, Onen F, Albrand G, et al. Pain tolerance and obstructive sleep apnea in the elderly. J Am Med Dir Assoc 2010;11:612–6.

25. Tarasiuk A, Greenberg-Dotan S, Simon-Tuval T, et al. The effect of obstructive sleep apnea on morbidity and health care utilization of middle-aged and older adults. J Am Geriatr Soc 2008;56:247–54.

26. Onen SH, Onen F, Courpron P, et al. How pain and analgesics disturb sleep. Clin J Pain 2005; 21:422–31.

27. Onen SH, Dubray C, Decullier E, et al. Observation-based nocturnal sleep inventory: screening tool for sleep apnea in elderly people. J Am Geriatr Soc 2008;56:1920–5.

28. Vitiello MV, Rybarczyk B, Von Korff M, et al. Cognitive behavioral therapy for insomnia improves sleep and decreases pain in older adults with co-morbid insomnia and osteoarthritis. J Clin Sleep Med 2009;5:355–62.

29. Ries LAG, Eisner MP, Kosary CL, et al. SEER cancer statistics review, 1973–1998. Bethesda (MD): National Institute of Health; 2000. NIH publication 00-2789.

30. Yancik R, Holmes ME. NIA/NCI Report of the Cancer Center Workshop (June 13–15, 2001). Exploring the role of cancer centers for integrating aging and cancer research. 2002. Available at: http://www.nia.nih.gov/ResearchInformation/ConferencesAndMeetings/WorkshopReport. Accessed October 25, 2016.

31. Palesh OG, Roscoe JA, Mustian KM, et al. Prevalence, demographics, and psychological associations of sleep disruption in patients with cancer. University of Rochester Cancer Center – Community Clinical Oncology Program. J Clin Oncol 2010;28: 292–8.

32. Davidson JR, MacLean AW, Brundage MD, et al. Sleep disturbance in cancer patients. Soc Sci Med 2002;54:1309–21.

33. Owen DC, Parker KP, McGuire DB. Comparison of subjective sleep quality in patients with cancer and healthy subjects. Oncol Nurs Forum 1999;26:1649–51.

34. Lee K, Cho M, Miaskowski C, et al. Impaired sleep and rhythms in persons with cancer. Sleep Med Rev 2004;8:199–212.

35. Roscoe JA, Kaufman ME, Matteson-Rusby SE, et al. Cancer related fatigue and sleep disorders. Oncologist 2007;12:35–42.

36. Engstrom CA, Strohl RA, Rose L, et al. Sleep alterations in cancer patients. Cancer Nurs 1999;22: 143–8.

37. Stiefel FC, Kornblith AB, Holland JC. Changes in the prescription patterns of psychotropic drugs for cancer patients during a 10-year period. Cancer 1990; 65:1048–53.

38. Derogatis LR, Feldstein M, Morrow G, et al. A survey of psychotropic drug prescriptions in an oncology population. Cancer 1979;44:1919–29.

39. O'Loughlin JL, Robitaille Y, Boivin JF, et al. Incidence of and risk factors for falls and injurious falls among the community-dwelling elderly. Am J Epidemiol 1993;137(3):342–54.

40. Tinetti ME, Doucette J, Claus E, et al. Risk factors for serious injury during falls by older persons in the community. J Am Geriatr Soc 1995;43:1214–21.

41. Carroll NV, Slattum PW, Cox FM. The cost of falls among the community-dwelling elderly. J Manag Care Pharm 2005;11(4):307–16.

42. Stone KL, Ewing SK, Lui LY, et al. Self-reported sleep and nap habits and risk of falls and fractures in older women: the study of osteoporotic fractures. J Am Geriatr Soc 2006;54:1177–83.

43. Helbig AK, Döring A, Heier M, et al. Association between sleep disturbances and falls among the elderly: results from the German Cooperative Health Research in the region of Augsburg-age study. Sleep Med 2013;14:1356–63.

44. Stone KL, Blackwell TL, Ancoli-Israel S, et al, Osteoporotic Fractures in Men Study Group. Sleep disturbances and risk of falls in older community-dwelling men: the outcomes of sleep disorders in older men (MrOS Sleep) study. J Am Geriatr Soc 2014;62: 299–305.

45. Glass J, Lanctôt KL, Herrmann N, et al. Sedative hypnotics in older people with insomnia: meta-analysis of risks and benefits. BMJ 2005; 331(7526):1169.

46. Avidan AY, Fries BE, James ML, et al. Insomnia and hypnotic use, recorded in the minimum data set, as predictors of falls and hip fractures in Michigan nursing homes. J Am Geriatr Soc 2005;53:955–62.

47. Latimer Hill E, Cumming RG, Lewis R, et al. Sleep disturbances and falls in older people. J Gerontol A Biol Sci Med Sci 2007;62(1):62–6.

48. Robillard R, Prince F, Filipini D, et al. Aging worsens the effects of sleep deprivation on postural control. PLoS One 2011;6:e28731.

49. Onen F, Higgins S, Onen SH. Falling-asleep–related injured falls in the elderly. J Am Med Dir Assoc 2009; 10:207–10.

50. Lloyd-Jones DM, Larson MG, Leip EP, et al. Lifetime risk for developing congestive heart failure-the

Framingham heart study. Circulation 2002;106: 3068–72.

51. McCullough PA, Philbin EF, Spertus JA, et al. Confirmation of a heart failure epidemic: findings from the Resource Utilization Among Congestive Heart Failure (REACH) study. J Am Coll Cardiol 2002;39:60–9.

52. Young T, Peppard PE, Gottlieb DJ. Epidemiology of obstructive sleep apnea: a population health perspective. Am J Respir Crit Care Med 2002;165: 1217–39.

53. Javaheri S, Parker TJ, Liming JD, et al. Sleep apnea in 81 ambulatory male patients with stable heart failure. Types and their prevalences, consequences, and presentations. Circulation 1998;97:2154–9.

54. Sin DD, Fitzgerald F, Parker JD, et al. Risk factors for central and obstructive sleep apnea in 450 men and women with congestive heart failure. Am J Respir Crit Care Med 1999;160(4):1101–6.

55. Lanfranchi PA, Braghiroli A, Bosimini E, et al. Prognostic value of nocturnal Cheyne-Stokes respiration in chronic heart failure. Circulation 1999;99: 1435–40.

56. Oldenburg O, Lamp B, Faber L, et al. Sleep-disordered breathing in patients with symptomatic heart failure: a contemporary study of prevalence in and characteristics of 700 patients. Eur J Heart Fail 2007;9:251–7.

57. Herrscher TE, Akre H, Overland B, et al. High prevalence of sleep apnea in heart failure outpatients:

even in patients with preserved systolic function. J Card Fail 2011;17:420–5.

58. Bitter T, Faber L, Hering D, et al. Sleep-disordered breathing in heart failure with normal left ventricular ejection fraction. Eur J Heart Fail 2009;11:602–8.

59. Yumino D, Redolfi S, Ruttanaumpawan P, et al. Nocturnal rostral fluid shift. A unifying concept for the pathogenesis of obstructive and central sleep apnea in men with heart failure. Circulation 2010; 121:1598–605.

60. Leung RS, Bradley TD. Sleep apnea and cardiovascular disease. Am J Respir Crit Care Med 2001; 164(12):2147–65.

61. Solin P, Kaye DM, Little PJ, et al. Impact of sleep apnea on sympathetic nervous system activity in heart failure. Chest 2003;123:1119–26.

62. Javaheri S, Javaheri S, Javaheri A. Sleep apnea, heart failure, and pulmonary hypertension. Curr Heart Fail Rep 2013;10:315–20.

63. Cowie MR, Woehrle H, Wegscheider K, et al. Adaptive servo-ventilation for central sleep apnea in systolic heart failure. N Engl J Med 2015;373:1095–105.

64. Netzer N, Ancoli-Israel S, Bliwise DL, et al. Principles of practice parameters for the treatment of sleep disordered breathing in the elderly and frail elderly: the consensus of the International Geriatric Sleep Medicine Task Force. Eur Respir J 2016;48: 992–1018.

Psychiatric Illness and Sleep in Older Adults
Comorbidity and Opportunities for Intervention

Michael R. Nadorff, PhD[a,b,*], Christopher W. Drapeau, PhD[a,c], Wilfred R. Pigeon, PhD[d,e]

KEYWORDS

- Sleep disorders • Psychiatric illness • Suicide • Older adults

KEY POINTS

- Sleep disorders are prevalent among older adults.
- Psychiatric disorders are highly comorbid with sleep disorders, though much less work has been conducted specifically examining older adults.
- Sleep disorders have been shown to be associated with suicide risk among older adults even beyond the effects of psychopathology.
- Research is needed to examine the potential for sleep interventions to improve both sleep and psychopathology symptoms among older adults.

Psychopathology is common among older adults, with community prevalence rates as high as 15% for anxiety[1] and 13% for depression.[2] Further, although in recent years suicide rates have been higher in midlife than among older adults, older white men still have the highest suicide rate of any group.[3] Although some may think that the onset of depression and anxiety among elders is understandable given the health and financial difficulties that may accompany aging, quality of life remains high. In fact, when external factors are controlled, age is not associated with quality of life.[4] Thus, the development of psychopathology, or suicidal behavior, in late life is *not* inevitable.

There is a great need for research examining what factors lead older adults to develop psychopathology. One area that has received increased attention of late is sleep disorders. Sleep disorders are highly prevalent among older adults, and many increase in prevalence as we age. For instance, insomnia has been found to be more prevalent among older adults than any other age group.[5] Further, although prevalent, insomnia may be underreported, as many older adults change their view of acceptable sleep or assume that they should not be able to sleep as well as they could when they were younger.[6,7] In addition to insomnia, many other sleep disorders become

This was not an industry-supported study, and the authors have no financial conflicts of interest.
Disclaimer: The views or opinions expressed herein do not reflect those of the Department of Veterans Affairs or the United States Government.
[a] Department of Psychology, Mississippi State University, PO Box 6161, Mississippi State, MS 39762, USA; [b] Menninger Department of Psychiatry and Behavioral Sciences, Baylor College of Medicine, 1977 Butler Boulevard, 4th Floor, Suite E4.100, Houston, TX 77030, USA; [c] Department of Education, Valparaiso University, 1800 Chapel Drive, Valparaiso, IN 46383, USA; [d] Department of Psychiatry, University of Rochester, Rochester, NY, USA; [e] VISN 2 Center of Excellence for Suicide Prevention, Canandaigua VA Medical Center, 400 Fort Hill Avenue, Canandaigua, NY 14424, USA
* Corresponding author. Department of Psychology, Mississippi State University, PO Box 6161, Mississippi, MS 39762.
E-mail address: mnadorff@psychology.msstate.edu

Sleep Med Clin 13 (2018) 81–91
https://doi.org/10.1016/j.jsmc.2017.09.008

more prevalent as we age, including obstructive sleep apnea,[8] restless leg syndrome,[9] and rapid eye movement (REM) sleep behavior disorder.[10] Lastly, although commonly thought of predominantly as a childhood disorder, research has demonstrated that nightmares can persist into late life.[11,12]

Although both psychopathology and sleep disturbances are prevalent among older adults, the extant literature examining their relation in older adulthood is not well developed. The present article reviews this literature, outlines areas where further research is necessary, and highlights opportunities for intervention.

SLEEP DISTURBANCES AND DISORDERS

From pain, to light, to things that go bump in the night, there are many factors that impact our sleep. Sleep disturbances include difficulty with initiating or maintaining sleep, waking too early, and dysfunctions that occur during sleep, such as sleepwalking or nightmares. The term *sleep disturbance* is used in a variety of manners. In its broadest usage, a sleep disturbance refers to any sleep problem, whether it is acute, chronic, or meets the diagnostic criteria as a sleep disorder. Here, the authors adopt the convention that sleep disturbances are problems with sleep commonly described as symptoms but that are not severe enough to be causing the individual significant impairment and/or to meet the diagnostic criteria for a sleep disorder. Once the individual is impaired and/or the symptoms associated with sleep disturbance are severe enough, then a sleep disorder diagnosis should be considered. Several classification manuals include sleep disorders, including the *International Classification of Diseases*,[13] the *Diagnostic and Statistical Manual of Mental Disorders*,[14] and the *International Classification of Sleep Disorders*.[15] There are 6 major categories of sleep disorders: insomnia, sleep-related breathing disorders, central disorders of hypersomnolence, circadian rhythm sleep-wake disorders, parasomnias, and sleep-related movement disorders.[15]

DEPRESSION AND SLEEP DISORDERS

Although depression is less prevalent among older adults than younger adults,[16] it is still a major concern for older adults, with approximately 13% to 15% prevalence in community samples.[2,17] Further, it is associated with decreased functioning and an increased risk of morbidity,[17] and more than half of all older adults who experience a depressive episode had their first episode 60

years of age or later.[18] Older adults who develop depression late in life are more likely to have vascular risk factors and cognitive deficits, whereas those who develop depression earlier are more likely to have a family history of depression and comorbid personality disorders.[17,19] Depression among older adults is more likely to present via physical complaints than affective complaints[20] and has higher rates of sleep complaints than depression in younger adults.[21] In fact, meta-analytic work has found that sleep disturbances more than double the risk of developing depression among older adults.[22]

Depression and Insomnia

Although commonly thought of as a symptom of depression,[14] numerous studies,[23–25] including those that focused on older adults,[26] have found that insomnia itself is a risk factor for developing depression (**Table 1**). Further, in the Improving Mood-Promoting Access to Collaborative Treatment (IMPACT) study, participants were between 1.8- and 3.5-times more likely to remain depressed than those who did not have insomnia.[27] The presence of insomnia also affects depression treatment, with less complete depressive symptom and suicidal ideation remission and higher rates of relapse in patients who have comorbid insomnia.[28,29] However, research on younger adults has found that adding cognitive-behavioral therapy (CBT) for insomnia to antidepressant treatment results in enhanced depression treatment outcomes.[30] Given this important finding, research examining the impact of treating insomnia on older adult depression treatment outcomes is warranted.

Depression and Obstructive Sleep Apnea

Obstructive sleep apnea (OSA) is a sleep-related breathing disorder characterized by excessive daytime sleepiness and frequent awakenings preceded by episodes whereby airflow is significantly reduced, or ceases entirely, despite the presence of respiratory effort.[15] The prevalence rates of OSA range dramatically (4%–50%) based on methodology, sex, and sample constitution; but epidemiologic studies all show an increase in prevalence rates with older age, with some plateauing within older age groups.[31–33] Results from mixed-sample studies of middle- and older-aged adults show that individuals with OSA often present with, or are at risk for developing, medical comorbidities (eg, cardiovascular disease, obesity) and have reductions in physical functioning and quality and frequency of social interactions, each of which can contribute to the onset or

Table 1
Summary of psychiatric illness, suicide, and sleep disorder research in older adults

	Insomnia	OSA	Nightmares	Sleep Quality
Depression	Insomnia symptoms increase the likelihood of depressive symptom onset and maintenance; there is a poor response to depression treatment.	No studies have targeted older adults specifically in regard to the prevalence of depression in OSA and the impact of CPAP adherence on remission of depressive symptoms.	Nightmares are strongly related to depressive symptoms. There is a lack of research replicating this finding and exploring the impact of nightmares on depression treatment outcomes.	Sleep quality predicts the onset and recurrence of depressive symptoms. The relationship seems stronger for men and those with earlier onset of depression (ie, 60–74 y).
Anxiety	Insomnia symptoms often co-occur with GAD and panic disorder. Alcohol consumption may moderate the association between insomnia symptoms and GAD. Anxiety symptoms may precede insomnia symptom onset.	Similar to depression, no studies have targeted older adults specifically in regard to the prevalence of anxiety in OSA and the impact of CPAP adherence on remission of anxious symptoms.	About 17% of those with significant anxiety report nightmares. Those with GAD report more bad dreams than those without GAD. Receiving CBT for anxiety may lead to fewer bad dreams after treatment and throughout the ensuing year.	
Suicide	Insomnia symptoms prospectively predict suicide across cultures. Depressive symptoms mediate the relation between insomnia symptoms and suicide ideation. Suicide attempt history is associated with more severe insomnia symptoms.	Suicide ideation has been reported among adults and older adults with OSA. CPAP adherence may be related to a remission of suicide-related thoughts. No studies have investigated for relationships between OSA and suicide risk.	The association between nightmares and suicide ideation is mediated by insomnia symptoms. The nightmare duration is independently related to suicide risk, even when controlling for insomnia symptoms.	Poor sleep quality prospectively predicts a fatal suicide attempt when controlling for depression (1.2-times greater risk).

Abbreviations: CBT, cognitive-behavioral therapy; CPAP, continuous positive airway pressure; GAD, generalized anxiety disorder; OSA, obstructive sleep apnea.

exacerbation of depression.[34,35] Greater OSA severity has been associated with the presence of depressive disorders,[36] and one study of Veterans Health Administration patients with OSA (N = 118,105; more than 38% were 65 years or older) estimated the prevalence of depression to be 21.8%.[37] There exists, however, a definitive and accessible intervention for OSA (ie, continuous positive airway pressure [CPAP]) that has been identified as the standard of care[38] and has been associated with decreases in depressive signs and symptoms among adult patients with OSA.[39–41] Given the prevalence of both depression and OSA in the general population, and their heightened prevalence in older cohorts, the relatively small number of studies at their intersection is somewhat striking.

Depression and Nightmares

Numerous studies of younger adults and mixed-age samples[42] have demonstrated a relation between nightmares and depressive symptoms, especially melancholic features of depression,[43] with some showing that the relation between depression and nightmares is independent of the effects of insomnia.[44] The few studies that have been conducted on nightmares and depression in older adults have shown a significant relationship between depressive symptoms and nightmares[11,45] and bad dream frequency.[12] In fact, the correlation between nightmares and depressive symptoms among older adults ($r = 0.70$)[11] is substantially higher than the correlation found among younger adults ($r = 0.33$).[46] Although this is based on very few studies, it is suggestive that nightmares are strongly related to depressive symptoms among older adults.

Although research has demonstrated a relation between nightmares and depression in older adults, it has yet to examine the impact of nightmares on the treatment of depression. Given the findings that insomnia symptoms are associated with poorer depression treatment outcomes,[28] and the strong relation between nightmares and depression among older adults,[11] research examining whether nightmares negatively affect depression treatment, particularly among older adults, is warranted.

Depression and Sleep Quality

Although not a sleep disorder per se, poor sleep quality has been found to prospectively predict both the onset and recurrence of depression in older adults.[47–49] Interestingly, the association between sleep disturbances and depression seems to be moderated by sex and age at depression onset.

Research has demonstrated that the relation between sleep quality and depression is stronger among men than women.[50] Additionally, adults with very late depression onset (aged 75 years or older) report fewer sleep disturbances than either those aged 18 to 59 years or 60 to 74 years.[51] Based on these findings, it seems that the relation between depression and sleep quality may be especially important for men up until 75 years of age.

ANXIETY AND SLEEP DISORDERS

Anxiety disorders are very common among older adults, with prevalence estimates as high as 14%.[52] Sleep disturbances are common in anxiety,[53] with daytime sleepiness, poor sleep quality, long sleep latency, and extended wake after sleep onset being common sleep complaints among those with anxiety.[54,55] In a sample of 2759 older adults aged 65 years and older, a sleep latency greater than 30 minutes was associated with a greater likelihood of meeting the criteria for an anxiety disorder and a decreased likelihood of meeting the criteria for a mood disorder.[56]

Anxiety and Insomnia

Anxiety and insomnia are commonly comorbid among older adults.[5] Specifically, insomnia has been found to commonly co-occur with panic disorder and generalized anxiety disorder (GAD).[57] Within a sample of older adults with GAD, more than 90% reported sleep dissatisfaction and 52% to 68% reported moderate to severe symptoms of insomnia.[58] It has been proposed that, in contrast to depression, anxiety likely precedes the development of insomnia[59] or both develop concurrently.[25]

Overall, the relation between insomnia and anxiety has been found to be very robust, with a large cross-sectional study finding that anxiety symptoms were associated with poorer sleep efficiency and greater sleep fragmentation after controlling for depressive symptoms, medical conditions, and antianxiety medication use.[60] However, one factor that has been shown to affect the relation is alcohol consumption. Surprisingly, mild to moderate drinking of alcohol seems to serve a protective function in older adults with GAD, as those who drank alcohol more often during the week had lower levels of anxiety, worry, and insomnia.[49,61]

Although the literature consistently shows that anxiety is associated with insomnia, there is still much we do not know. Anxiety is a very broad area that encompasses several disorders. Further research is necessary in order to understand how each anxiety disorder is associated with insomnia and how they may differ in this regard.

Anxiety and Obstructive Sleep Apnea

Few studies have focused on exploring for the relationships between OSA and anxiety among older adults. In fact, a recent review of the general research literature concluded that the relation between OSA and anxiety continues to be poorly illustrated.[62] At present, the literature is mixed, with some studies showing the prevalence of anxiety among individuals with OSA as high as 70%,[63] whereas others have found no relation between the severity of apnea symptoms and anxiety symptoms.[64] Thus, there is a great need for more research in this understudied area to help us better understand whether sleep apnea is associated with anxiety across the adult life span. Also, and similar to depression, relatively few studies have examined the impact of CPAP adherence on anxiety in older adults with OSA; but decreases in anxious symptoms have been observed among adult patients with OSA.[48]

Anxiety and Nightmares

Despite research demonstrating that 17% of older adults with clinically significant symptoms of anxiety experience nightmares,[65] as opposed to 4% prevalence for older adults without anxiety,[66] few studies have examined this relation. One of the few studies that has been conducted examined bad dreams within the context of late life GAD, finding that older adults with GAD endorsed significantly more bad dreams than those without GAD. Further, the frequency of bad dreams was associated with greater worry, poorer quality of life, and increased symptoms of anxiety and depression.[12] However, these effects may be mitigated through CBT for anxiety. Older adults who received CBT for anxiety reported fewer bad dreams at post-treatment as well as throughout a year of follow-up.[12]

SUICIDE AND SLEEP DISORDERS

Older adults, but especially Caucasian older adult men, are at an elevated risk of suicide.[3] There are now 2 meta-analyses and several review articles confirming an association between sleep disturbance and/or specific sleep disorders and suicide outcomes, such as suicidal ideation, nonfatal suicide attempts, and death by suicide.[67–70]

Late-life suicide is also associated with some key demographic risk factors that may overlap with factors related to late-life sleep disorders. For example, the 2015 US suicide rates indicate a notable increase in the number of women aged 45 to 64 years who died by suicide when compared with 1999 data, with a similar though less dramatic increase among women aged 65 to 74 years. Whereas women's risk peaks in midlife, men's risk continues to be highest after 75 years of age.[3] The baby boom cohort, which has had relatively higher rates of suicide across the life cycle when compared with other birth cohorts, is beginning to leave the middle years and enter older adulthood in increasingly large numbers each year. This change is likely to have a pronounced effect on the incidence and prevalence of both sleep disorders and suicide in older adults.

Suicide and Insomnia

The relation between insomnia and suicide has been well examined among younger adults, and several studies have been conducted in older adults. One study measuring sleep quality in older adults showed that poor sleep at baseline significantly predicted death by suicide when controlling for depression.[71] The same research team recently completed a case-control cohort study of older adults showing that poor subjective sleep at baseline was associated with a 1.2-times greater risk for a fatal suicide attempt by the 10-year follow up, even when controlling for depressive symptoms.[72] Additionally, difficulty falling asleep was associated with a 2.24-times greater suicide risk, and nonrestorative sleep was associated with a 2.17-times greater risk for suicide.[72] This finding mirrors studies that have taken place outside the United States, where insomnia has been prospectively linked with suicide among Taiwanese older adults[73] and in an epidemiologic survey of Chinese older adults,[74] suggesting these findings may generalize across cultures.

There have also been cross-sectional studies that have examined the relation between insomnia and suicidal risk among older adults. In a sample of older adults recruited from a community medicine clinic, insomnia symptoms were found to be related to suicide ideation, even when controlling for nightmares, though the relation was mediated by depressive symptoms.[11] Additionally, a recent study found that participants with a history of a suicide attempt had more severe insomnia symptoms than those with depression or suicidal ideation, even when controlling for demographics, past month alcohol abuse, cognitive ability, depression severity, anxiety, and perceived physical health burden.[75] Thus, there is consensus in the literature that insomnia is associated with suicide risk among older adults. However, it is not clear whether treating insomnia reduces suicide risk; future research investigating this important question would be of great value to the literature.

Suicide and Nightmares

Although a small literature, there is evidence that nightmares are associated with suicide.[11,45] Among a sample of older adults recruited from a primary care clinic, nightmares were found to be associated with suicidal ideation, though this relation was mediated by insomnia symptoms.[11] However, recent research suggests that the duration of time that one has had nightmares may be more important than how severe their symptoms are currently. In a sample of older adults recruited through Amazon's Mechanical Turk, Golding and colleagues[45] found that the nightmare duration was associated with suicide risk independent of current symptoms of insomnia, nightmares, anhedonia, and feelings of burdensomeness and lack of belongingness. There is a great need for additional studies investigating this relation in order to determine whether the nightmare duration should be considered a risk factor for suicide among older adults as well as whether treating nightmares may ameliorate the consequences of long-term nightmares.

Suicide and Obstructive Sleep Apnea

As noted earlier, beyond increasing the overall disease burden, the presence of OSA-related comorbidities can contribute to depression. Not surprisingly, these factors are also associated with a greater risk of suicide.[76,77] Nonetheless, only 2 published observational studies[78,79] and one case study[80] have examined the relation between OSA and suicidality; only 2 of the 3 included older adults.[78,80] Among 228 patients with OSA who adhered to CPAP treatment (31% older than 65 years of age), 18% endorsed suicide ideation before treatment and none endorsed thoughts of suicide at the 3-month follow-up.[78] In addition, a significant decreases in depression and OSA severity were observed following 3 months of CPAP. Similarly, a remission of suicide-related thoughts in a 74-year-old man adhering to nasal CPAP was outlined in the case study.[80]

Two of the 3 studies that examined the relationship between suicide risk and OSA relied on single items to assess suicidal ideation, and only one used objective sleep measures.[79] The lack of research concerning the relationship between OSA and suicidality is an important gap to address.

NEURODEGENERATIVE DISEASES AND SLEEP DISORDERS
Rapid Eye Movement Sleep Behavior Disorder and Parkinson Disease

Parkinson disease (PD) is a prevalent neurodegenerative disease in late life that results in cognitive

impairment ranging from mild cognitive impairment through dementia.[81] It is also closely related to dementia with Lewy bodies, a related dopaminergic disorder that is the second most common type of degenerative dementia.[82] REM sleep behavior disorder (RSBD), a parasomnia whereby there is an absence of full atonia and paralysis during REM sleep resulting in the individual acting out his or her dreams,[83] is commonly comorbid with PD (**Table 2**). Further, it is debated in the literature whether RSBD may either be a prodromal symptom of PD[84] or part of a distinct clinical entity.[85] Proponents of RSBD being a prodromal symptom of PD point to research demonstrating that patients with idiopathic RSBD have up to a 72% chance of developing PD[86] and an 80% risk of developing a neurodegenerative synucleinopathy.[84] Further, patients with RSBD evidence basal ganglia dysfunction similar to patients with early stage PD.[87] However, those arguing for a different clinical entity cite research that when RSBD precedes PD, there is no difference in the clinical presentation of the patients with PD; but when RSBD comes after PD, patients with PD had worse PD symptoms and required higher doses of dopaminergic agonists.[85] Additionally, on autopsy, those who have both PD and RSBD showed more synuclein pathology than those who just had PD.[88] Regardless of this debate, the literature is in strong agreement regarding the relation between RSBD and PD.

Sleep in Dementia

Sleep disturbances are very common in dementia, with patients with dementia having significantly lower sleep efficiency and more time awake throughout the night.[89] Because patients with dementia are commonly awake and requiring care, these sleep disturbances are often one of the most distressing symptoms to caregivers of patients with dementia.[90] A recent review of the literature on sleep disorders and cognitive decline[91] found that sleep disorders significantly impact both physical and cognitive functioning as well as behavior problems among those with cognitive decline and dementia. Thus, in addition to being distressing to caregivers, sleep disorders may worsen the symptoms of cognitive impairment and dementia. Research has also suggested that OSA may increase the risk of cognitive impairment and dementia.[92] Additionally, prospective research found that both a short ($\leq$6 hours) and long (>9 hours) time in bed is associated with an increased risk of developing dementia at follow-up.[93,94]

Although there is a strong literature suggesting an association between dementia and sleep

Table 2
Summary of neurodegenerative diseases and sleep disorder research in older adults

	RSBD		Sleep Disturbance	Sleep Disorders
PD	RSBD and PD often co-occur. Patients with idiopathic RSBD have an increased risk of developing PD and a neurodegenerative synucleinopathy. Those diagnosed with RSBD following a diagnosis of PD display worse PD symptoms than those with only PD.	Dementia	Reduced sleep efficiency and more time awake throughout the night are common in dementia. Time in bed prospectively predicts the development of dementia (ie, 6 h and less or more than 9 h).	Sleep disorders impact both cognitive and physical functioning. OSA may increase the cognitive impairment risk.

disturbances, relatively little work has been done on sleep interventions among individuals with dementia.[95] Cognitive therapies may not be appropriate due to cognitive impairments, and research has suggested that benzodiazepine medications also are not appropriate[96,97] nor effective[98] for individuals with dementia. Thus, there is a great need for research investigating sleep treatments for individuals with dementia. In particular, given the strong association between OSA and cognitive difficulties, apnea should be treated when possible.[97] Further, behavioral interventions to improve sleep quality may be an especially strong fit and are worthy of investigation.

SUMMARY
Summary of Findings and Conclusions

Although the late-life literature is still in its infancy compared with the literature on younger adults, the literature that exists consistently shows concurrence with the broader literature that psychopathology is highly comorbid with sleep disturbances in late life. That said, there are some notable differences between the older and younger adults. First, although psychopathology is prevalent in late life, the rates of psychopathology are lower among older adults than they are in young adulthood.[17] On the other hand, with some exceptions, such as nightmares,[99] sleep disturbances are more prevalent among older adults than they are earlier in the life span.[100] Thus, although we see a correlation between sleep disturbances and psychopathology across the life span, the strength of the association may change with age. A good example of this is the relation between insomnia symptoms, nightmares, and suicidal ideation. Among young adults, research has demonstrated that nightmares, but not insomnia

symptoms, are associated with suicidal ideation independent of each other.[42] However, among older adults we find that insomnia symptoms are associated with suicidal ideation independent of nightmares.[11] Given this, there is a need for further research extending the sleep and psychopathology findings from young adult and mixed-age samples to older adults.

Another area that is particularly promising and warrants further research is examining the impact of treating sleep disorders on psychopathology in older adults. Research in mixed-age samples has shown that for many forms of psychopathology treatment may be enhanced through the addition of sleep interventions. However, relatively little research in this vein has been done among older adults. Relatedly, although much of the early work providing evidence of efficacy of behavioral insomnia interventions was undertaken in older adults, there is a need for further research on sleep interventions among older adults with psychiatric comorbidities. It is often difficult to treat sleep problems among older adults because of cognitive and memory problems, which may interfere with CBT.

In conclusion, although research on the relationship of sleep difficulties and psychopathology among older adults lags in comparison with the work in younger populations, it is clear that there is an association between sleep disturbances and psychopathology across a spectrum of psychiatric disorders in older adults. This association provides an opportunity to intervene in sleep problems to potentially reduce the development or exacerbation of psychopathology as people age. It is also plausible that the efficacy of interventions to treat psychiatric disorders can be enhanced by addressing the sleep complaints that may be playing an important role behind the scenes.

REFERENCES

1. Bryant C, Jackson H, Ames D. The prevalence of anxiety in older adults: methodological issues and a review of the literature. J Affect Disord 2008; 109(3):233–50.
2. Laborde-Lahoz P, El-Gabalawy R, Kinley J, et al. Subsyndromal depression among older adults in the USA: prevalence, comorbidity, and risk for new-onset psychiatric disorders in late life. Int J Geriatr Psychiatry 2015;30(7): 677–85.
3. Centers for Disease Control and Prevention. Web-based injury statistics query and reporting system. n.d. Available at: http://www.cdc.gov/injury/wisqars/index.html. Accessed February 7, 2017.
4. Netuveli G, Blane D. Quality of life in older ages. Br Med Bull 2008;85(1):113–26.
5. Thase ME. Correlates and consequences of chronic insomnia. Gen Hosp Psychiatry 2005; 27(2):100–12.
6. Vitiello MV, Larsen LH, Moe KE. Age-related sleep change: gender and estrogen effects on the subjective-objective sleep quality relationships of healthy, noncomplaining older men and women. J Psychosom Res 2004;56(5):503–10.
7. Leger D, Poursain B. An international survey of insomnia: under-recognition and under-treatment of a polysymptomatic condition. Curr Med Res Opin 2005;21(11):1785–92.
8. Norman D, Loredo JS. Obstructive sleep apnea in older adults. Clin Geriatr Med 2008;24(1):151.
9. Kim WH, Kim BS, Kim SK, et al. Restless legs syndrome in older people: a community-based study on its prevalence and association with major depressive disorder in older Korean adults. Int J Geriatr Psychiatry 2012;27(6):565–72.
10. Ju Y-E, Larson-Prior L, Duntley S. Changing demographics in REM sleep behavior disorder: possible effect of autoimmunity and antidepressants. Sleep Med 2011;12(3):278–83.
11. Nadorff MR, Fiske A, Sperry JA, et al. Insomnia symptoms, nightmares and suicidal ideation in older adults. J Gerontol B Psychol Sci Soc Sci 2013;68(2):145–52.
12. Nadorff MR, Porter B, Rhoades HM, et al. Bad dream frequency in older adults with generalized anxiety disorder: prevalence, correlates, and effect of cognitive behavioral treatment for anxiety. Behav Sleep Med 2014;12(1):28–40.
13. World Health Organization. International statistical classification of diseases and related health problems. 10th edition. Geneva, Switzerland: World Health Organization; 2007.
14. American Psychiatric Association. Diagnostic and statistical manual of mental disorders, 5th edition. 5th edition. Washington, DC: Author; 2013.
15. American Academy of Sleep Medicine. International classification of sleep disorders. 3rd edition. Chicago: American Academy of Sleep Medicine; 2014.
16. Hasin DS, Goodwin RD, Stinson FS, et al. Epidemiology of major depressive disorder: results from the National Epidemiologic Survey on Alcoholism and related conditions. Arch Gen Psychiatry 2005; 62(10):1097–106.
17. Fiske A, Wetherell JL, Gatz M. Depression in older adults. Annu Rev Clin Psychol 2009;5:363–89.
18. Brodaty H, Luscombe G, Parker G, et al. Early and late onset depression in old age: different aetiologies, same phenomenology. J Affect Disord 2001;66(2–3):225–36.
19. Schweitzer I, Tuckwell V, O'Brien J, et al. Is late onset depression a prodrome to dementia? Int J Geriatr Psychiatry 2002;17(11):997–1005.
20. Gallo JJ, Anthony JC, Muthen BO. Age differences in the symptoms of depression: a latent trait analysis. J Gerontol 1994;49(6):P251–64.
21. Christensen H, Jorm AF, Mackinnon AJ, et al. Age differences in depression and anxiety symptoms: a structural equation modelling analysis of data from a general population sample. Psychol Med 1999;29(2):325–39.
22. Cole MG, Dendukuri N. Risk factors for depression among elderly community subjects: a systematic review and meta-analysis. Am J Psychiatry 2003; 160(6):1147–56.
23. Baglioni C, Battagliese G, Feige B, et al. Insomnia as a predictor of depression: a meta-analytic evaluation of longitudinal epidemiological studies. J Affect Disord 2011;135(1–3):10–9.
24. Baglioni C, Riemann D. Is chronic insomnia a precursor to major depression? Epidemiological and biological findings. Curr Psychiatry Rep 2012; 14(5):511–8.
25. Ohayon MM, Roth T. Place of chronic insomnia in the course of depressive and anxiety disorders. J Psychiatr Res 2003;37(1):9–15.
26. Perlis ML, Smith LJ, Lyness JM, et al. Insomnia as a risk factor for onset of depression in the elderly. Behav Sleep Med 2006;4(2):104–13.
27. Pigeon WR, Hegel M, Unützer J, et al. Is insomnia a perpetuating factor for late-life depression in the IMPACT cohort? Sleep 2008; 31(4):481–8.
28. Taylor DJ, Walters HM, Vittengl JR, et al. Which depressive symptoms remain after response to cognitive therapy of depression and predict relapse and recurrence? J Affect Disord 2009; 123(1–3):181–7.
29. Nadorff MR, Ellis TE, Allen JG, et al. Presence and persistence of sleep-related symptoms and suicidal ideation in psychiatric inpatients. Crisis 2014;35(6):398–405.

30. Manber R, Edinger JD, Gress JL, et al. Cognitive behavioral therapy for insomnia enhances depression outcome in patients with comorbid major depressive disorder and insomnia. Sleep 2008; 31(4):489–95.

31. Young T, Evans L, Finn L, et al. Estimation of the clinically diagnosed proportion of sleep apnea syndrome in middle-aged men and women. Sleep 1997;20(9):705–6.

32. Alexander M, Ray MA, Hebert JR, et al. The National Veteran Sleep Disorder Study: descriptive epidemiology and secular trends, 2000-2010. Sleep 2016;39(7):1399–410.

33. Franklin KA, Lindberg E. Obstructive sleep apnea is a common disorder in the population-a review on the epidemiology of sleep apnea. J Thorac Dis 2015;7(8):1311–22.

34. Akashiba T, Kawahara S, Akahoshi T, et al. Relationship between quality of life and mood or depression in patients with severe obstructive sleep apnea syndrome. Chest 2002;122(3):861–5.

35. Yang EH, Hla KM, McHorney CA, et al. Sleep apnea and quality of life. Sleep 2000;23(4):535–41.

36. Schröder CM, O'Hara R. Depression and obstructive sleep apnea (OSA). Ann Gen Psychiatry 2005;4:13.

37. Sharafkhaneh A, Giray N, Richardson P, et al. Association of psychiatric disorders and sleep apnea in a large cohort. Sleep 2005;28(11):1405–11.

38. Epstein LJ, Kristo D, Strollo PJ Jr, et al. Clinical guideline for the evaluation, management and long-term care of obstructive sleep apnea in adults. J Clin Sleep Med 2009;5(3):263–76.

39. Millman RP, Fogel BS, McNamara ME, et al. Depression as a manifestation of obstructive sleep apnea: reversal with nasal continuous positive airway pressure. J Clin Psychiatry 1989;50(9): 348–51.

40. Borak J, Cieslicki J, Szelenberger W, et al. Psychopathological characteristics of the consequences of obstructive sleep apnea prior to and 3 months after therapy. Psychiatr Pol 1993;27(1):43–55 [in Polish].

41. Sanchez AI, Buela-Casal G, Bermudez MP, et al. The effects of continuous positive air pressure treatment on anxiety and depression levels in apnea patients. Psychiatry Clin Neurosci 2001;55(6): 641–6.

42. Nadorff MR, Nazem S, Fiske A. Insomnia symptoms, nightmares, and suicidal ideation in a college student sample. Sleep 2011;34(1):93–8.

43. Agargun MY, Besiroglu L, Cilli AS, et al. Nightmares, suicide attempts, and melancholic features in patients with unipolar major depression. J Affect Disord 2007;98(3):267–70.

44. Nakajima S, Inoue Y, Sasai T, et al. Impact of frequency of nightmares comorbid with insomnia on depression in Japanese rural community residents: a cross-sectional study. Sleep Med 2014;15(3): 371–4.

45. Golding S, Nadorff MR, Winer ES, et al. Unpacking sleep and suicide in older adults in a combined online sample. J Clin Sleep Med 2015;11(12):1385–92.

46. Nadorff MR, Nazem S, Fiske A. Insomnia symptoms, nightmares, and suicide risk: duration of sleep disturbance matters. Suicide Life Threat Behav 2013;43(2):139–49.

47. Cho HJ, Lavretsky H, Olmstead R, et al. Sleep disturbance and depression recurrence in community-dwelling older adults: a prospective study. Am J Psychiatry 2008;165(12):1543–50.

48. Lee E, Cho HJ, Olmstead R, et al. Persistent sleep disturbance: a risk factor for recurrent depression in community-dwelling older adults. Sleep 2013; 36(11):1685–91.

49. Jaussent I, Dauvilliers Y, Ancelin M-L, et al. Insomnia symptoms in older adults: associated factors and gender differences. Am J Geriatr Psychiatry 2011;19(1):88–97.

50. Schechtman KB, Kutner NG, Wallace RB, et al. Gender, self-reported depressive symptoms, and sleep disturbance among older community-dwelling persons. J Psychosom Res 1997;43(5): 513–27.

51. Corruble E, Gorwood P, Falissard B. Association between age of onset and symptom profiles of late-life depression. Acta Psychiatr Scand 2008; 118(5):389–94.

52. Wolitzky-Taylor KB, Castriotta N, Lenze EJ, et al. Anxiety disorders in older adults: a comprehensive review. Depress Anxiety 2010;27(2):190–211.

53. Wetherell JL, Le Roux H, Gatz M. DSM-IV criteria for generalized anxiety disorder in older adults: distinguishing the worried from the well. Psychol Aging 2003;18(3):622–7.

54. Potvin O, Lorrain D, Belleville G, et al. Subjective sleep characteristics associated with anxiety and depression in older adults: a population-based study. Int J Geriatr Psychiatry 2014;29(12): 1262–70.

55. Yu J, Rawtaer I, Fam J, et al. Sleep correlates of depression and anxiety in an elderly Asian population. Psychogeriatrics 2016;16(3):191–5.

56. Leblanc M-F, Desjardins S, Desgagné A. Sleep problems in anxious and depressive older adults. Psychol Res Behav Manag 2015;8:161–9.

57. Ohayon MM, Roth T. What are the contributing factors for insomnia in the general population? J Psychosom Res 2001;51(6):745–55.

58. Brenes GA, Miller ME, Stanley MA, et al. Insomnia in older adults with generalized anxiety disorder. Am J Geriatr Psychiatry 2009;17(6): 465–72.

59. Johnson EO, Roth T, Breslau N. The association of insomnia with anxiety disorders and depression: exploration of the direction of risk. J Psychiatr Res 2006;40(8):700–8.

60. Spira AP, Stone K, Beaudreau SA, et al. Anxiety symptoms and objectively measured sleep quality in older women. Am J Geriatr Psychiatry 2009; 17(2):136–43.

61. Ivan MC, Amspoker AB, Nadorff MR, et al. Alcohol use, anxiety, and insomnia in older adults with generalized anxiety disorder. Am J Geriatr Psychiatry 2014;22(9):875–83.

62. Diaz SV, Brown LK. Relationships between obstructive sleep apnea and anxiety. Curr Opin Pulm Med 2016;22(6):563–9.

63. Saunamaki T, Jehkonen M. Depression and anxiety in obstructive sleep apnea syndrome: a review. Acta Neurol Scand 2007;116(5):277–88.

64. Asghari A, Mohammadi F, Kamrava SK, et al. Severity of depression and anxiety in obstructive sleep apnea syndrome. Eur Arch Otorhinolaryngol 2012;269(12):2549–53.

65. Mallon L, Broman J-E, Hetta J. Sleeping difficulties in relation to depression and anxiety in elderly adults. Nord J Psychiatry 2000;54(5):355–60.

66. Salvio M-A, Wood JM, Schwartz J, et al. Nightmare prevalence in the healthy elderly. Psychol Aging 1992;7(2):324–5.

67. Pigeon WR, Pinquart M, Conner K. Meta-analysis of sleep disturbance and suicidal thoughts and behaviors. J Clin Psychiatry 2012;73(9):e1160–7.

68. Malik S, Kanwar A, Sim LA, et al. The association between sleep disturbances and suicidal behaviors in patients with psychiatric diagnoses: a systematic review and meta-analysis. Syst Rev 2014; 3:18.

69. Bernert RA, Kim JS, Iwata NG, et al. Sleep disturbances as an evidence-based suicide risk factor. Curr Psychiatry Rep 2015;17(3):554.

70. Bernert RA, Nadorff MR. Sleep disturbances and suicide risk. Sleep Med Clin 2015;10(1):35–9.

71. Bernert R, Turvey C, Conwell Y, et al. Sleep disturbance as a unique risk factor for completed suicide. Sleep 2007;30:A344.

72. Bernert RA, Turvey CL, Conwell Y, et al. Association of poor subjective sleep quality with risk for death by suicide during a 10-year period: a longitudinal, population-based study of late life. JAMA Psychiatry 2014;71(10):1129–37.

73. Hung GC, Kwok CL, Yip PS, et al. Predicting suicide in older adults - a community-based cohort study in Taipei City, Taiwan. J Affect Disord 2015; 172:165–70.

74. Chiu HFK, Dai J, Xiang YT, et al. Suicidal thoughts and behaviours in older adults in rural China: a preliminary study. Int J Geriatr Psychiatry 2012;27(11): 1124–30.

75. Kay DB, Dombrovski AY, Buysse DJ, et al. Insomnia is associated with suicide attempt in middle-aged and older adults with depression. Int Psychogeriatr 2016;28(4):613–9.

76. Fanning JR, Pietrzak RH. Suicidality among older male veterans in the United States: results from the National Health and Resilience in Veterans Study. J Psychiatr Res 2013;47(11):1766–75.

77. Thompson JM, Zamorski MA, Sweet J, et al. Roles of physical and mental health in suicidal ideation in Canadian Armed Forces Regular Force veterans. Can J Public Health 2014;105(2):e109–15.

78. Edwards C, Mukherjee S, Simpson L, et al. Depressive symptoms before and after treatment of obstructive sleep apnea in men and women. J Clin Sleep Med 2015;11(9):1029–38.

79. Krakow B, Artar A, Warner TD, et al. Sleep disorder, depression and suicidality in female sexual assault survivors. Crisis 2000;21(4):163–70.

80. Krahn LE, Miller BW, Bergstrom LR. Rapid resolution of intense suicidal ideation after treatment of severe obstructive sleep apnea. J Clin Sleep Med 2008;4(1):64–5.

81. Janvin CC, Larsen JP, Aarsland D, et al. Subtypes of mild cognitive impairment in Parkinson's disease: progression to dementia. Mov Disord 2006; 21(9):1343–9.

82. Donaghy PC, McKeith IG. The clinical characteristics of dementia with Lewy bodies and a consideration of prodromal diagnosis. Alzheimers Res Ther 2014;6(4):46.

83. Nadorff MR, Rose MW. Parasomnias. The encyclopedia of clinical psychology. Hoboken (NJ): John Wiley & Sons, Inc; 2014.

84. Postuma RB. Prodromal Parkinson's disease – using REM sleep behavior disorder as a window. Parkinsonism Relat Disord 2014;20(Suppl 1):S1–4.

85. Ferri R, Cosentino FII, Pizza F, et al. The timing between REM sleep behavior disorder and Parkinson's disease. Sleep Breath 2014;18(2):319–23.

86. Kim YE, Jeon BS. Clinical implication of REM sleep behavior disorder in Parkinson's disease. J Parkinsons Dis 2014;4(2):237–44.

87. Rolinski M, Griffanti L, Piccini P, et al. Basal ganglia dysfunction in idiopathic REM sleep behaviour disorder parallels that in early Parkinson's disease. Brain 2016;139(8):2224–34.

88. Postuma RB, Adler CH, Dugger BN, et al. REM sleep behavior disorder and neuropathology in Parkinson's disease. Mov Disord 2015;30(10): 1413–7.

89. Kume Y, Kodama A, Sato K, et al. Sleep/awake status throughout the night and circadian motor activity patterns in older nursing-home residents with or without dementia, and older community-dwelling people without dementia. Int Psychogeriatr 2016; 28(12):2001–8.

90. Nozoe KT, Polesel DN, Jeronimo G, et al. Sleep disturbance in people with dementia and its effect on caregivers. Australas J Ageing 2015;34(4): 277–8.

91. Guarnieri B, Sorbi S. Sleep and cognitive decline: a strong bidirectional relationship. It is time for specific recommendations on routine assessment and the management of sleep disorders in patients with mild cognitive impairment and dementia. Eur Neurol 2015;74(1–2):43–8.

92. Buratti L, Luzzi S, Petrelli C, et al. Obstructive sleep apnea syndrome: an emerging risk factor for dementia. CNS Neurol Disord Drug Targets 2016; 15(6):678–82.

93. Bokenberger K, Ström P, Dahl Aslan AK, et al. Association between sleep characteristics and incident dementia accounting for baseline cognitive status: a prospective population-based study. J Gerontol A Biol Sci Med Sci 2017;72(1):134–9.

94. Chen J-C, Espeland MA, Brunner RL, et al. Sleep duration, cognitive decline, and dementia risk in older women. Alzheimers Dement 2016;12(1): 21–33.

95. Cipriani G, Lucetti C, Danti S, et al. Sleep disturbances and dementia. Psychogeriatrics 2015; 15(1):65–74.

96. Schutte-Rodin S, Broch L, Buysse D, et al. Clinical guideline for the evaluation and management of chronic insomnia in adults. J Clin Sleep Med 2008;4(5):487–504.

97. Ooms S, Ju Y-E. Treatment of sleep disorders in dementia. Curr Treat Options Neurol 2016;18(9):40.

98. Brown DT, Westbury JL, Schüz B. Sleep and agitation in nursing home residents with and without dementia. Int Psychogeriatr 2015;27(12): 1945–55.

99. Nadorff MR, Nadorff DK, Germain A. Nightmares: under-reported, undetected, and therefore untreated. J Clin Sleep Med 2015;11(7):747–50.

100. Ohayon MM. Epidemiology of insomnia: what we know and what we still need to learn. Sleep Med Rev 2002;6(2):97–111.

Sleep and Cognition in Older Adults

Joseph M. Dzierzewski, PhD[a],*, Natalie Dautovich, PhD[b], Scott Ravyts, MS[c]

KEYWORDS

- Sleep • Insomnia • Sleep apnea • Cognition • Cognitive function • Age • Aging

KEY POINTS

- Sleep and cognitive functioning both show negative changes with advanced age.
- Although the relationships are uncertain, sleep seems to be related to cognitive functioning within good-sleeping older adults, older adults with insomnia, and older adults with sleep disordered breathing.
- Both insomnia and sleep apnea may be associated with cognitive decline and dementia.
- Treatment of sleep disorders may provide cognitive benefits in late life. Additional research is warranted.

INTRODUCTION

This article reviews the growing literature examining sleep and cognitive functioning in older adults. The main focus is on normal, age-related cognitive changes, as opposed to neurodegenerative disease processes. Age-related cognitive changes are the result of developmental maturation. These cumulative, long-term processes are universal or nearly universal, and are resistant to efforts to reverse the change.[1,2] Investigation into cognitive aging has found a general cognitive decline experienced with increasing age,[3–5] which has been shown to be pervasive, affecting many subdomains of cognition, including:

- Reaction time
- Sensory processing
- Attention
- Memory
- Reasoning
- Executive functioning

Although much is known regarding developmental changes in cognitive functioning, comparatively little is known regarding sleep's relationship to late-life cognitive functioning.

Sleep represents an intriguing individual difference variable because it may relate to late-life cognitive functioning. Sleep has shown consistent age-related changes as a result of developmental maturation. Many of these developmental changes parallel the age-related changes observed in cognitive functioning. For example, slow wave sleep (stage N3) and rapid eye movement (REM) sleep both decrease with advanced age.[6] In addition to these normal, developmentally appropriate changes in sleep, older adults also experience an increased prevalence of both insomnia and sleep disordered breathing (SDB).[7–9] **Fig. 1** shows general age-related changes in cognitive functioning and general age-related changes in sleep. The parallel changes in sleep and cognition with age, coupled

Disclosure: Dr J.M. Dzierzewski was supported by a grant from the National Institute on Aging (K23AG049955). Dr N. Dautovich serves as a sleep consultant for the National Sleep Foundation and Merck Sharp & Dohme Corp. S. Ravyts reports no commercial or financial conflicts of interest.
[a] Department of Psychology, Virginia Commonwealth University, 806 West Franklin Street, Room 306, Box 842018, Richmond, VA 23284-2018, USA; [b] Department of Psychology, Virginia Commonwealth University, 800 West Franklin Street, Room 203, Box 842018, Richmond, VA 23284-2018, USA; [c] Department of Psychology, Virginia Commonwealth University, Box 842018, Richmond, VA 23284-2018, USA
* Corresponding author.
E-mail address: dzierzewski@vcu.edu

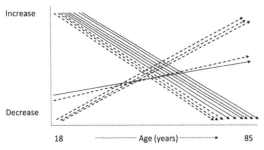

Increase

Decrease

18 ——————— Age (years)————→ 85

Fig. 1. Normative changes with age in both cognitive functioning and sleep. Solid arrows represent general cognitive changes. Dashed arrows represent general sleep changes. Cognitive abilities that decline with age include processing speed, working memory, long-term memory, attention, reasoning, and executive control. Sleep characteristics that decline with age include total sleep time, slow wave sleep, and REM sleep. Sleep characteristics that increase with age include wake time after sleep onset, and light sleep (stages N1 and N2). Crystalized intelligence and sleep onset latency both showed slight increases with advancing age.

with anecdotal reports of disturbed cognitive abilities following poor sleep, have resulted in research efforts focused on examining sleep and cognition in older adults. This article summarizes the literature for normal-sleeping older adults, older adults with insomnia, and older adults with SDB.

SLEEP AND COGNITION IN NORMAL-SLEEPING OLDER ADULTS
Self-Reported Sleep Duration and Cognition

Several large-scale epidemiologic studies have garnered information regarding habitual sleep duration and/or difficulty and cognitive functioning in older adults. In a study of more than 3000 older adults, long sleep duration was associated with worse overall/global cognitive functioning, whereas no association with short sleep duration and cognitive functioning was observed.[10] In a similar study of more than 5000 adults, sleep duration was associated with verbal fluency and list memory, such that both long and short sleep durations were associated with poorer performance.[11] In a sample of community-dwelling older women, sleeping less than 5 hours per night was associated with poorer global cognition and poorer performance across many of the individual indicators of cognitive functioning (ie, verbal memory, verbal fluency, working memory) compared with women sleeping 7 hours or more per night.[12] The investigators of these studies suggest that sleep duration may be related to cognitive

functioning through changes in sleep architecture, fragmentation, quality, and neurologic conditions.[10,11] The relationship between self-reported retrospective recall of habitual sleep duration and cognitive functioning has been confirmed through meta-analysis showing deleterious effects in both long and short sleepers on multiple domains of cognitive functioning in older adults.[13]

Polysomnography-Measured Sleep and Cognition

Investigation into the relationship between polysomnography (PSG)-assessed sleep and waking cognitive functioning has provided mixed results. It has been reported that longer sleep onset latency is related to poorer verbal memory and executive functioning, whereas greater total wake time is related to lower psychomotor speed and memory in normal-sleeping older adults.[13] However, in another investigation, slow wave sleep was unrelated to performance on a simple reaction time task, continuous performance task, and attention test in good-sleeping older adults.[14] As such, it seems that additional research is need to further explicate the relationship between PSG-measured sleep and cognitive functioning in older adults without a sleep complaint.

Actigraphy-Measured Sleep and Cognition

It seems that there is a relationship between objective, naturally occurring sleep measured with actigraphy and cognitive performance. In a study of nearly 3000 older community-dwelling women, actigraphy-measured sleep (sleep efficiency, sleep onset latency, wake after sleep onset, and napping) was associated with an increased risk of poorer general cognition and executive performance.[15] However, total sleep time was not related to cognitive functioning, which led the investigators to conclude that "it is disturbance of sleep rather than quantity that affects cognition."[15] In a different but complementary vein, 7 nights of actigraphy were used to compute sleep/wake patterns in 144 community-dwelling older adults. Older adults who displayed many shifts from rest to activity performed worse on composites of executive functioning, memory, and speed than elderly with more consistent rest-activity patterns.[16] The scarcity of research examining actigraphy-measured sleep and cognition in older adults precludes any definitive conclusions being drawn.

Sleep Deprivation and Cognition

In general, short-term total sleep deprivation has a significant deleterious effect across most cognitive domains, including attention, working memory, processing speed, short-term memory, and reasoning, with smaller effects being observed for tasks of greater complexity.[17] Webb and Levy[18] and Webb[19] conducted experiments to examine potential age differences in cognitive response to sleep deprivation. In both experiments, older adults' and younger adults' performance on a variety of cognitive tasks were compared following 2 nights of sleep deprivation. Older adults showed greater deterioration following sleep deprivation than did the younger adults in vigilance, visual search, reaction times, word detection, addition, anagrams, and objects uses.[18,19] Jones and Harrison[20] summarized the extant sleep deprivation work by stating that, "neurocognitive studies present many inconsistencies, task classification is often ambiguous and, in the absence of any unifying explanation at the level of cognitive mechanisms, the overall picture is one of a disparate range of impairment following sleep loss."[20]

Sleep Restriction and Cognition

Bliese and colleagues[21] examined age-related changes in reaction time/attention after modest sleep restriction. Older adults showed less pronounced effects of sleep restriction on their reaction times than younger adults. However, the oldest adult included in the study was 62 years old, so aging effects must be interpreted cautiously. Nevertheless, the investigators suggest that older adults may have "expended more effort across days"[21] so this could have resulted in blunted differences. The experimental evidence regarding the sleep-cognition relationship gained through studies using sleep restriction methodology have consistently yielded results indicating an impact on vigilance, which may be blunted in older adults.[21] Regarding potential mechanisms underlying the relationship between sleep restriction and cognitive functioning, Banks and Dinges[22] summarized the evidence by suggesting that there is no "definitive evidence of what is accumulating and destabilizing cognitive functions over time when sleep is regularly restricted."[22]

Sleep and Learning

As opposed to examination of the negative consequences of poor sleep (or sleep loss), some researchers have investigated the potential benefits of sleep gained. In this line of research, participants are allowed to sleep while manipulating the timing of cognitive testing/training to either allow sleep to occur following testing or not in order to examine any effects of posttraining

sleep on subsequent testing. Most of this research has been conducted with younger adults, and with findings indicating optimized performance following sleep. Tucker and colleagues[23] trained 16 healthy older adults in a finger tapping sequencing task and found that older adults performed significantly better following sleep than 12 hours of not sleeping, suggesting sleep-dependent motor skill performance in the elderly. Older adults showed similar rates of improvement as were found in younger samples; however, specific sleep characteristics did not correlate with the next day's performance (in contrast, stage 2 sleep and sleep spindle activity does correlate in younger adults). The investigators concluded that sleep in the elderly does optimize motor skill learning; however, it may do so differently than in younger adults.[23]

SLEEP AND COGNITION IN OLDER ADULTS WITH INSOMNIA

Older adults are at an increased risk for both insomnia and experiencing negative changes in cognitive functioning. Given the comorbidity of insomnia and cognitive dysfunction in older adults, researchers have attempted to understand the role of insomnia in predicting cognitive functioning in a variety of samples (eg, cognitively intact older adults and older adults experiencing cognitive decline or dementia). Furthermore, a small number of studies have examined the effect of behavioral interventions for insomnia on cognitive outcomes. A sample of representative studies is presented later that illustrates these different approaches.

Insomnia Status and Normal Cognitive Aging

The association between insomnia and cognitive performance in younger and middle-aged adults is well established, with impairments in working memory, episodic memory, and some aspects of executive functioning.[24] However, less is known about the association between insomnia diagnosis and cognitive performance in cognitively healthy older adults who are not experiencing cognitive decline or dementia. To date, insomnia and cognitive functioning have been examined in older adults with insomnia through cross-sectional designs with matched healthy controls[25,26] or using comparisons across insomnia subtypes.[27]

Overall, in contrast with healthy controls, insomnia status was associated with worse performance on a subset of cognitive tasks. Specifically, participants with insomnia performed significantly worse on memory span, integration of visual and semantic dimensions, and executive functioning tasks.[26] The insomnia groups performed better than healthy controls on the simple attending task.[25] The better attentional performance on simple attending did not persist for complex attending, perhaps reflecting the higher arousal that is characteristic of individuals diagnosed with insomnia.[28] This higher arousal may be beneficial for unambiguous stimuli but a hindrance for complex tasks requiring more cognitive resources.[25] In addition to differences in cognitive performance dependent on the presence or absence of insomnia, performance also seems to differ depending on the type of insomnia complaint. Specifically, Ling and colleagues[27] found that only early morning awakening was associated with significantly worse cognitive performance in the executive functioning domain. No association was found between difficulty initiating sleep or difficulty maintaining sleep across the following cognitive domains: attention, verbal memory, visuospatial ability, and executive functioning. **Table 1** lists the differences in cognitive functioning between older adults with and without insomnia.

Overall, across the reviewed studies examining cognitive performance in cognitively intact older adults with insomnia, insomnia status and specific characteristics of insomnia (eg, early morning awakening) seem to be associated with worse cognitive performance. However, the poorer performance of the individuals with insomnia is not consistent across all cognitive domains or across all tasks within cognitive domains. Consequently, despite a trend toward worse cognitive performance associated with insomnia status, the existing body of evidence is too small and inconsistent to arrive at a broad conclusion.

Insomnia and Cognitive Decline/Dementia Diagnoses

Compared with research that has examined insomnia and cognitive performance in cognitively healthy older adults, more work has been done to explore the role of insomnia in predicting cognitive decline or dementia status. Despite the greater breadth of research with cognitively impaired older adults, the association between insomnia and cognitive decline and/or dementia status remains unclear.

A minority of studies identified a negative association between insomnia and cognitive decline or dementia.[29,30] Specifically, older adults with long-term insomnia and long-term use of hypnotics had a 2-fold risk of developing dementia during a 3-year follow-up period compared with healthy controls.[29] Controlling for hypnotic use, similar results were found with long-term insomnia predicting an increased risk for cognitive decline at a 3-year follow-up for older adults with insomnia compared with healthy controls.[30] These results point to the importance of considering the duration of the insomnia complaint as a predictor of cognitive function, because long-term, rather than concurrent, sleep complaint was associated with cognitive decline.[30]

In contrast, another subsection of studies found a positive association between insomnia symptoms and cognitive performance.[31,32] Using a longitudinal design, Jaussent and colleagues[31] (2012) found that complaints of awakenings during the night and total number of insomnia complaints at baseline predicted a decreased risk for cognitive decline during an 8-year follow-up period. In addition, a cross-sectional approach with older adults with dementia residing in assisted living facilities showed that individuals with insomnia symptoms performed significantly better on the Mini-Mental State Examination (MMSE) than those without insomnia symptoms.[32] Of note, neither of these studies assessed the duration of the insomnia complaint.

Despite a subset of studies showing negative and positive associations between insomnia and

Table 1
Differences in performance across cognitive tasks group by insomnia status

Cognitive Task	Better Performance by Insomnia Group	Better Performance by Healthy Control Group	No Group Difference
Sustained attention	X (simple tasks)[25]	X (simple tasks,[26] complex tasks[25])	X (complex tasks)[26]
Naming	—	—	X[26]
Psychomotor skills	—	—	X[26]
Memory span	—	X[26]	—
Integration of 2 dimensions (visual and semantic)	—	X[26]	—
Time estimation	—	X[26]	—
Executive functioning	—	X[26]	—

cognitive decline or dementia, a greater number of studies have found no association. Using longitudinal and cross-sectional designs, with and without comparison groups, and various approaches to insomnia and cognitive evaluations, insomnia was not associated with cognitive decline[33–35] or dementia status in many studies.[36] Given these discrepant findings, it could be concluded that insomnia status does not predict cognitive decline in older adults. However, it is more likely that the equivocal findings result from methodological differences in research approaches. **Table 2** provides a summary of the relationship between insomnia and cognitive decline/dementia status in older adults.

Insomnia Treatment and Cognitive Functioning

In addition to examining cross-sectional and longitudinal associations between insomnia and cognitive outcomes, a small number of studies have investigated whether the treatment of insomnia leads to an improvement in cognitive performance (**Table 3**).[25,37] In one such study, an insomnia intervention was used with community-dwelling older adults with insomnia.[25] The insomnia intervention consisted of sleep restriction, cognitive restructuring, sleep hygiene, bright light exposure, body temperature manipulations, and structured physical activity. Following treatment, sleep onset latency and sleep efficiency were significantly improved in the treatment group compared with the waitlist group. Treatment was also associated with improved performance on complex vigilance tasks and worsened performance on simple vigilance tasks compared with the waitlist control. A possible explanation for the performance differences on simple versus complex tasks following treatment is that improved sleep results in a reduction of arousal levels to normal,[25] resulting in slower performance on simpler tasks.

An additional study used a brief behavioral treatment of insomnia approach with a sample of community-dwelling older adults who were cognitively intact and diagnosed with insomnia.[37] Individuals in the treatment group showed a significantly greater decrease in wake time after sleep onset following treatment compared with the information-only control group. However, the treatment group did not show significantly better improvement in cognitive performance across 3 cognitive domains (episodic memory, working memory, abstract reasoning) compared with the control group. The investigators posited that the null findings might be caused by the short follow-up period (4 weeks after the start of the intervention). Allowing more time postintervention for the sleep treatment to take effect might have enabled detection of effects on cognitive performance.

SLEEP AND COGNITION IN OLDER ADULTS WITH SLEEP DISORDERED BREATHING

The estimated prevalence of both SDB and cognitive impairment increases with age.[38,39] Moreover, individuals with SDB show cognitive changes similar to those associated with aging.[40] Recent research has posited that SDB and advanced age act independently to impair cognitive functioning, with the combination of both SDB and advanced age leading to cognitive impairments greater than either factor alone.[40]

Although some studies have found an association between SDB and impairments in global cognitive functioning,[41,42] not all cognitive domains seem to be equally affected. Instead, the domains of vigilance, executive function, and memory are particularly implicated.[43] The impact of SDB on all 3 of these cognitive domains has been observed among both community-based and clinic-based populations with different neuropsychological tests (**Table 4**). SDB in older adults has been found to impair:

- Vigilance[44,45]
- Attention[46–49]
- Reaction time[50]
- Executive functioning[47,51,52]
- Problem solving[53]
- Verbal recall[52,54,55]
- Nonverbal recall[53]
- Episodic memory[51]

Although few studies have examined the longitudinal impact of SDB on cognitive performance in older adults, preliminary evidence suggests that SDB can contribute to relevant long-term changes. For example, one study found that SDB was associated with a decline in global cognitive functioning over 3 years.[41] Similarly, another study of community-dwelling adults found that SDB was associated with a decline in attention abilities over 8 years.[48]

The long-term impact of SDB may also influence the onset and course of certain neurologic disorders. Individuals with SDB have higher rates of both mild cognitive impairment and dementia at an earlier age.[56,57] Evidence also suggests that older adults with neurologic disorders might be more vulnerable to the negative cognitive effects of SDB.[45] For example, SDB can exacerbate cognitive impairments in older adults with dementia.[58] The possible role of SDB in the development

Table 2
Insomnia status and cognitive decline or dementia diagnosis

Insomnia Measure	Cognitive Measure	Results	Study
Negative Associations			
ICD-9 codes	ICD-9 codes	Patients with insomnia diagnosis and prescribed hypnotics, > risk for dementia during the 3-y follow-up compared with controls	29
Interview indicating either problem most of the time: trouble falling asleep or waking up too early and not falling asleep again	Pfeiffer's SPMSQ, ≥2 errors on the SPMSQ classified as cognitive decline	Insomnia associated with increased risk of cognitive decline for men, independent of depression and comorbid with depression. Insomnia associated with increased risk of cognitive decline for women when insomnia was comorbid with depression	30
Positive Associations			
Interview and questionnaire: difficulty initiating sleep, awakenings during the night, early morning awakening, insomnia severity	Incident cognitive impairment defined as 4-point reduction in MMSE, 4-point reduction in BVRT, and 14-point reduction in the IST scores	Number of insomnia complaints and difficulty with awakenings during the night were negatively associated with MMSE cognitive decline during follow-up. No associations found for BVRT or IST	31
Johns Hopkins Alzheimer's Disease Research Center questionnaire	Severity of dementia was classified based on MMSE scores (mild = MMSE >20; moderate = MMSE 11–19; severe = MMSE <10)	Participants diagnosed with insomnia performed better on the MMSE than those without sleep disturbance or those with insomnia and daytime sleepiness	32
No Associations			
Self-report questionnaire assessing "Usually having trouble falling asleep or waking up far too early and not going back to sleep"	CASI; cognitive decline was defined as a ≥9-point decrease in the CASI	Insomnia not associated with greater risk for dementia diagnosis or cognitive decline	33

Interview assessing difficulty falling asleep, staying asleep, or both	Incident cognitive impairment defined as an MMSE ≤21	No sleep problems associated with increased risk for incident cognitive impairment at 2 and 10 year follow-ups	34
Clinical interview: at least 1 symptom (difficulty falling asleep, staying asleep, early morning awakening) occurring at least 3 times a week	MMSE; Global Deterioration Scale. Participants with MMSE <24.0 were evaluated for dementia by expert panel	Insomnia diagnosis was not associated with cognitive impairment	35
Insomnia Interview Schedule and Sleep Impairment Index: onset, maintenance, termination insomnia	Alzheimer disease diagnosis was made according to NINCDS/ADRDA and DSM-IV criteria	Individuals with Alzheimer disease did not differ from the healthy comparison group in terms of the frequency of onset, maintenance, termination of insomnia symptoms	36

Abbreviations: ADRDA, Alzheimer's Disease and Related Disorders Association; BVRT, Benton Visual Retention Test; CASI, cognitive abilities screening instrument; DSM-IV, diagnostic and statistical manual of mental disorders, fourth edition; ICD-9, International Classification of Diseases, Ninth Revision; IST, Isaacs Set Test; MMSE, Mini-Mental State Examination; NINCDS, National Institute of Neurological Disorders and Stroke; SPMSQ, short portable mental status questionnaire.

Table 3
Insomnia treatment and cognitive performance

Insomnia Measure	Cognitive Measure	Results	Study
DSM-IV criteria, Pittsburgh Sleep Quality Index, Sleep Disorders Questionnaire. PSG and sleep diaries were also used	Simple and complex sustained attention assessed via computer. Outcomes: lapses, false-positive responses, and reaction times	Compared with the waitlist control, insomnia intervention group showed increased reaction time for simple vigilance task and reduced reaction time for complex vigilance task	25
DSM-IV-TR, ICSD-2 verified by self-report questionnaires and clinical interview. Polysomnography and the Pittsburgh Sleep Quality Index were also used	Neuropsychological tests assessed 3 cognitive domains: episodic memory, working memory, abstract reasoning	Insomnia intervention was not associated with greater improved cognitive performance compared with information-only control	37

Abbreviations: DSM-IV-TR, DSM-IV text revision; ICSD-2, International Classification of Sleep Disorders, second edition.

of neurologic disorders has led researchers to examine the possible pathways contributing to impairments in cognitive functioning.

Several mechanisms through which SDB contributes to cognitive decline in older adults have been proposed. Evidence suggests that high levels of hypoxemia, an abnormally low level of oxygen in the blood, may play a prominent role. Yaffe and colleagues[57] found that hypoxemia was associated with an increased risk of future mild cognitive impairment and dementia. In addition, increased hypoxemia is associated with greater impairment in global cognitive functioning, as well as declines in specific cognitive domains.[44,59] However, other studies have found no association between hypoxemia and impaired cognition.[41,55] As a result, both sleep fragmentation and excessive daytime sleepiness have been proposed as alternative mechanisms through which SDB may lead to cognitive dysfunction.[60] For example, excessive daytime sleepiness caused by SDB was associated with a decline in global cognitive functioning.[41] Despite these findings, the relative contributions of both sleep fragmentation and excessive daytime sleepiness to cognitive impairment remain poorly understood.

Although strong evidence supports an association between SDB and cognitive decline in older adults, not all findings support this association. One study found that although both SDB and aging are independently associated with cognitive deficits, age did not interact with SDB to make those cognitive deficits worse.[61] Other studies report similar findings. Boland and colleagues[62] found no evidence for an association between either mild or moderate forms of SDB and

cognitive functioning in verbal learning and short-term recall, psychomotor efficiency, or verbal fluency. Similarly, other research found no association between SDB and performance on broad standardized cognitive tests.[63,64] Studies that found no association between SDB and cognitive impairment in older adults contain several methodological differences. First, they lacked comprehensive measures of cognitive functioning or relied on single measures of global functioning.[62] Cognitive impairments in older adults with SDB may be subtle and may not be readily identified by general/global cognitive measures. Second, several of the studies that found no association between SDB and cognition used homePSG,[64] which has been shown to differ from laboratory PSG, particularly for adults with severe SDB.[65] In addition, several studies finding no associations between SDB and cognitive performance only included participants with mild to moderate SDB,[62,63] suggestive of a dose-response relationship between SDB severity and cognitive performance.

Although the findings are inconsistent, overall, current research suggests that SDB adversely affects cognitive performance in older adults. Cognitive impairments are particularly pronounced in the domains of attention, executive function, and memory. These findings are largely consistent with research examining the influence of SDB in young and middle-aged adults.[66,67]

Sleep Disordered Breathing Severity and Cognitive Performance

Research has explored whether the severity of SDB (as indexed by the apnea-hypopnea index

Table 4
Cognitive performance in older adults with sleep disordered breathing

Cognitive Domain	Measures	Outcomes	Representative References
Global functioning	• MMSE	• EDS is associated with global cognitive decline over 3 y • Increased levels of hypoxemia and AHI are associated with lower global cognition functioning	41,42
Vigilance	• Digital Vigilance Test • Psychomotor Vigilance Test • Trail-making Test Part A • Digit Symbol Substitution/Coding Subtest • Vienna Test System	• SDB is associated with decreased vigilance • Increased hypoxemia is associated with decreased vigilance • Increased RDI is associated with decreased attention • Older adults with SDB have slower reaction times compared with age-match controls and younger adults	44,45,49,50
Executive function	• Stroop Color and Word Test • Trail-making Test Part B • Similarities Subtest • Raven Progressive Matrices	• Higher RDI associated with decreased executive function • RDI associated with lower cerebral efficiency • SDB is associated with a greater decline of executive function over time • Severe SDB is associated with poorer executive functioning • SDB is associated with poorer problem-solving abilities	47,49,51,52
Memory	• Hopkins Verbal Learning Test • Brief Visuospatial Memory Test–Revised • Rey Auditory Verbal Learning Test	• SDB is associated with lower nonverbal delayed recall • Increased AHI and RDI are associated with decreased verbal delayed recall memory • Severe SDB is associated with poorer episodic memory over time	53–55

Abbreviations: AHI, apnea-hypopnea index; EDS, excessive daytime sleepiness; RDI, respiratory disturbance index.

[AHI] or respiratory disturbance index [RDI]) is related to the level of cognitive impairment in older adults. Studies have found that greater AHI and RDI were associated with poorer global cognitive functioning,[42] as well as adverse outcomes on specific cognitive domains such as:

• Vigilance[45,48,68]
• Executive functioning[52]
• Language functioning[69]
• Attention[47,49]
• Executive function[47,49]
• Memory[54]

However, one study examining older adults with mostly mild to moderate SDB found no association between SDB severity and cognitive functioning,[62] suggesting that there may be a threshold at which SDB exerts an increasingly negative impact on cognition. Further research investigating SDB severity and cognitive impairment is warranted.

Sleep Disordered Breathing Treatment and Cognitive Performance

Given the nature of cognitive dysfunction in older adults with SDB, as well as the association between SDB and neurologic disorders, the influence of SDB treatment on cognitive functioning in older adults has been the subject of recent interest. The most common treatment of SDB is positive airway pressure (PAP) therapy. Although PAP has been shown to decrease some of the primary sequelae of SDB, such as sleep fragmentation and nocturnal oxygen saturation, several studies suggest possible benefits of PAP treatment on cognitive performance.

Two studies report improvements in many areas of cognitive functioning following 3 months of PAP treatment.[54,70] Improvements were shown in the following domains:

- Episodic memory
- Short-term memory
- Executive functioning
- Attention
- Psychomotor speed
- Nonverbal delayed recall

Despite optimism about the potential benefits of PAP on cognition, some studies have shown more limited and uneven benefits of PAP treatment. For example, Kang and colleagues[71] found that short-term PAP treatment was associated with gains in executive functioning but no other cognitive domains.

Preliminary evidence suggests that cognitive gains observed with short-term PAP treatment might be maintained over time. PAP treatment over the course of 10 years is associated with better memory, attention, and executive functioning.[51] The long-term benefits of PAP treatment may also extend to older adults with neurologic disorders. Preliminary examination of long-term PAP use among individuals with Alzheimer disease found that treatment can slow cognitive deterioration.[72] Another recent study reported that PAP treatment may delay the age of onset of mild cognitive impairment.[56]

Although the influence of PAP treatment on cognitive outcomes seems promising, noncompliance with the treatment remains prevalent in the general population, as well as among older adults.[73] Limited compliance may severely limit the benefits of PAP treatment on cognitive abilities. Older adults who complied with treatment (average use of 8.5 hours per night) showed greater cognitive abilities compared with individuals who were noncompliant (3.9 hours per night).[54] One hypothesis about PAP compliance is that older adults who notice cognitive gains in readily observable domains, such as attention and memory, may be more likely to comply with PAP treatment.[54]

Although preliminary evidence shows improved cognitive outcomes for older adults treated with PAP, further research is needed to confirm these findings and better understand which cognitive domains are affected. In addition, future research

Table 5
Theories on the link between sleep and cognition

Name	Description	Reference
Controlled attention	Monotonous tasks are most affected by sleep loss because of the amount of top-down control needed to sustain attention, whereas more complex/difficult tasks are intrinsically motivating (ie, bottom-up control)	31
Neuropsychological	Sleep loss results in focal impairment in functions subserved by the prefrontal cortex (ie, executive functions), beyond any impairment in attention or vigilance	17,20,75
Vigilance/arousal	Attention, which is needed for the performance of many other cognitive tasks, is mediated by arousal; a common correlated feature of disturbed sleep	76,77
Wake-state instability	Cognitive deficits observed as a result of sleep loss occur because of the interaction of the drive to maintain alertness and the homeostatic drive to initiate sleep	78–80

Please note that these theories are not mutually exclusive but attempt to explain similar phenomena in different ways.

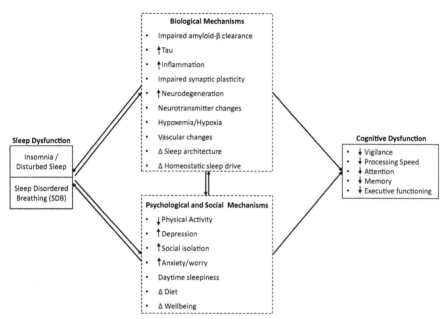

Fig. 2. Model depicting the relationships between (1) insomnia/disturbed sleep, (2) sleep disordered breathing and cognitive functioning in older adults. Factors listed in dashed boxes represent potential biopsychosocial mechanisms through which sleep may impact cognitive functioning.

should examine whether other forms of SDB treatment, such as weight loss, oral appliance therapy, positional therapy, and surgical treatments, might lead to similar cognitive gains.

UNIFYING THEORIES AND MECHANISMS

There are several informative hypotheses concerning sleep and cognitive functioning. These hypotheses include the controlled attention hypothesis,[74] neuropsychological hypothesis,[17,20,75] vigilance/arousal hypothesis,[76,77] and wake-state instability hypothesis.[78–80] These various theories about the role of sleep processes in regulating and maintaining cognitive functioning may not be mutually exclusive.[17] The controlled attention and vigilance/arousal hypotheses are essentially parallel descriptions of the same phenomenon. Many higher order cognitive functions may rely on the appropriate levels of attention and arousal. It has been suggested that impairment of the prefrontal cortex may cause decrements in attention and vigilance.[81] Sleep seems to impede arousal/vigilance/attention and prefrontal functioning, potentially through instability of the neurobiological systems responsible for attentional and sleep drives. **Table 5** provides a description of each sleep-cognition theory. In addition to the sleep-cognition hypotheses discussed earlier, there are many suspected mechanisms involved in the sleep-cognition relationship in late life. These mechanisms are graphically depicted in **Fig. 2**.

SUMMARY AND FUTURE DIRECTIONS

Sleep and cognitive functioning seem to be related in late life; however, the exact nature of this relationship has yet to be discerned. Future studies should continue to investigate the gamut of sleep-cognition relationships. Important questions remain concerning (1) the role of normal sleep changes in normal cognitive aging; (2) the role of pathologic sleep changes in the development of dementias; and (3) the utility of treating sleep disorders for improving cognitive functioning, warding off unwanted cognitive decline, and slowing the course of neurodegenerative diseases. An intriguing prospect for future study is to examine the additive impact of treating sleep disorders in conjunction with focused cognitive interventions. Perhaps the combination of interventions that focus on different pathways of change may have a synergistic effect and result in more pronounced cognitive improvements. Increasing knowledge of the ways in which sleep may affect late-life cognitive functioning could have far-reaching benefits.

REFERENCES

1. Li S-C, Huxhold O, Schmiedek F. Aging and attenuated processing robustness. Gerontology 2003; 50(1):28–34.
2. Nesselroade JR. The warp and the woof of the developmental fabric. In: Downs RM, Liben LS,

Palermo DS, editors. Visions of aesthetics, the environment & development: the legacy of Joachim F. Wohlwill. Hillsdale (NJ): Lawrence Erlbaum Associates; 1991. p. 213–40.

3. Park DC, Smith AD, Lautenschlager G, et al. Mediators of long-term memory performance across the life span. Psychol Aging 1996;11(4):621.

4. Schaie KW, Willis SL, Caskie GI. The Seattle longitudinal study: relationship between personality and cognition. Neuropsychol Dev Cogn B Aging Neuropsychol Cogn 2004;11(2–3):304–24.

5. Salthouse TA. What and when of cognitive aging. Curr Dir Psychol Sci 2004;13(4):140–4.

6. Morgan K. Sleep and aging. In: Lichstein K, Morin C, editors. Treatment of late-life insomnia. Thousand Oaks (CA): Sage Publications; 2000. p. 3–36.

7. Foley DJ, Monjan AA, Brown SL, et al. Sleep complaints among elderly persons - an epidemiological study of 3 communities. Sleep 1995;18:425–32.

8. Newman AB, Enright PL, Manolio TA, et al. Sleep disturbance, psychosocial correlates, and cardiovascular disease in 5201 older adults: the Cardiovascular Health Study. J Am Geriatr Soc 1997; 45(1):1–7.

9. Young T, Peppard PE, Gottlieb DJ. Epidemiology of obstructive sleep apnea: a population health perspective. Am J Respir Crit Care Med 2002; 165(9):1217–39.

10. Faubel R, López-García E, Guallar-castillÓn P, et al. Usual sleep duration and cognitive function in older adults in Spain. J Sleep Res 2009;18(4):427–35.

11. Kronholm E, Sallinen M, Suutama T, et al. Self-reported sleep duration and cognitive functioning in the general population. J Sleep Res 2009;18(4): 436–46.

12. Tworoger SS, Lee S, Schernhammer ES, et al. The association of self-reported sleep duration, difficulty sleeping, and snoring with cognitive function in older women. Alzheimer Dis Assoc Disord 2006; 20(1):41–8.

13. Bastien CH, Fortier-Brochu É, Rioux I, et al. Cognitive performance and sleep quality in the elderly suffering from chronic insomnia: relationship between objective and subjective measures. J Psychosom Res 2003;54(1):39–49.

14. Crenshaw MC, Edinger JD. Slow-wave sleep and waking cognitive performance among older adults with and without insomnia complaints. Physiol Behav 1999;66(3):485–92.

15. Blackwell T, Yaffe K, Ancoli-Israel S, et al. Poor sleep is associated with impaired cognitive function in older women: the study of osteoporotic fractures. J Gerontol A Biol Sci Med Sci 2006;61(4):405–10.

16. Oosterman JM, van Someren EJ, Vogels RL, et al. Fragmentation of the rest-activity rhythm correlates with age-related cognitive deficits. J Sleep Res 2009;18(1):129–35.

17. Lim J, Dinges DF. A meta-analysis of the impact of short-term sleep deprivation on cognitive variables. Psychol Bull 2010;136(3):375.

18. Webb WB, Levy CM. Age, sleep deprivation, and performance. Psychophysiology 1982;19(3):272–6.

19. Webb WB. A further analysis of age and sleep deprivation effects. Psychophysiology 1985;22(2):156–61.

20. Jones K, Harrison Y. Frontal lobe function, sleep loss and fragmented sleep. Sleep Med Rev 2001;5(6): 463–75.

21. Bliese PD, Wesensten NJ, Balkin TJ. Age and individual variability in performance during sleep restriction. J Sleep Res 2006;15(4):376–85.

22. Banks S, Dinges DF. Behavioral and physiological consequences of sleep restriction. J Clin Sleep Med 2007;3(5):519–28.

23. Tucker M, McKinley S, Stickgold R. Sleep optimizes motor skill in older adults. J Am Geriatr Soc 2011; 59(4):603–9.

24. Fortier-Brochu E, Beaulieu-Bonneau S, Ivers H, et al. Insomnia and daytime cognitive performance: a meta-analysis. Sleep Med Rev 2012;16(1):83–94.

25. Altena E, Van Der Werf YD, Strijers RLM, et al. Sleep loss affects vigilance: effects of chronic insomnia and sleep therapy. J Sleep Res 2008;17(3):335–43.

26. Haimov I, Hanuka E, Horowitz Y. Chronic insomnia and cognitive functioning among older adults. Behav Sleep Med 2008;6(1):32–54.

27. Ling A, Lim ML, Gwee X, et al. Insomnia and daytime neuropsychological test performance in older adults. Sleep Med 2016;17:7–12.

28. Nofzinger EA, Buysse DJ, Germain A, et al. Functional neuroimaging evidence for hyperarousal in insomnia. Am J Psychiatry 2004;161(11):2126–8.

29. Chen P-L, Lee W-J, Sun W-Z, et al. Risk of dementia in patients with insomnia and long-term use of hypnotics: a population-based retrospective cohort study. PLoS One 2012;7(11):e49113. Forloni G, editor.

30. Cricco M, Simonsick EM, Foley DJ. The impact of insomnia on cognitive functioning in older adults. J Am Geriatr Soc 2001;49(9):1185–9.

31. Jaussent I, Bouyer J, Ancelin M-L, et al. Excessive sleepiness is predictive of cognitive decline in the elderly. Sleep 2012;35(9):1201–7.

32. Rao V, Spiro J, Samus QM, et al. Insomnia and daytime sleepiness in people with dementia residing in assisted living: findings from the Maryland Assisted Living Study. Int J Geriatr Psychiatry 2008;23(2): 199–206.

33. Foley D, Monjan A, Masaki K, et al. Daytime sleepiness is associated with 3-year incident dementia and cognitive decline in older Japanese-American men. J Am Geriatr Soc 2001;49(12):1628–32.

34. Keage HAD, Banks S, Yang KL, et al. What sleep characteristics predict cognitive decline in the elderly? Sleep Med 2012;13(7):886–92.

35. Merlino G, Piani A, Gigli GL, et al. Daytime sleepiness is associated with dementia and cognitive decline in older Italian adults: a population-based study. Sleep Med 2010;11(4):372–7.

36. Ohadinia S, Noroozian M, Shahsavand S, et al. Evaluation of insomnia and daytime napping in Iranian Alzheimer disease patients: relationship with severity of dementia and comparison with normal adults. Am J Geriatr Psychiatry 2004; 12(5):517–22.

37. Wilckens KA, Hall MH, Nebes RD, et al. Changes in cognitive performance are associated with changes in sleep in older adults with insomnia. Behav Sleep Med 2016;14(3):295–310.

38. Peppard PE, Young T, Barnet JH, et al. Increased prevalence of sleep-disordered breathing in adults. Am J Epidemiol 2013;177(9):1006–14.

39. Hedden T, Gabrieli JD. Insights into the ageing mind: a view from cognitive neuroscience. Nat Rev Neurosci 2004;5(2):87–96.

40. Ayalon L, Ancoli-Israel S, Drummond SP. Obstructive sleep apnea and age: a double insult to brain function? Am J Respir Crit Care Med 2010;182(3): 413–9.

41. Cohen-Zion M, Stepnowsky C, Marler M, et al. Changes in cognitive function associated with sleep disordered breathing in older people. J Am Geriatr Soc 2001;49(12):1622–7.

42. Spira AP, Blackwell T, Stone KL, et al. Sleep-disordered breathing and cognition in older women. J Am Geriatr Soc 2008;56(1):45–50.

43. Zimmerman ME, Aloia MS. Sleep-disordered breathing and cognition in older adults. Curr Neurol Neurosci Rep 2012;12(5):537–46.

44. Blackwell T, Yaffe K, Ancoli-Israel S, et al. Associations between sleep architecture and sleep-disordered breathing and cognition in older community-dwelling men: the osteoporotic fractures in men sleep study. J Am Geriatr Soc 2011;59(12): 2217–25.

45. Kim H, Dinges DF, Young T. Sleep-disordered breathing and psychomotor vigilance in a community-based sample. Sleep 2007;30(10): 1309–16.

46. Dealberto MJ, Pajot N, Courbon D, et al. Breathing disorders during sleep and cognitive performance in an older community sample: the EVA study. J Am Geriatr Soc 1996;44(11):1287–94.

47. Hayward L, Mant A, Eyland A, et al. Sleep disordered breathing and cognitive function in a retirement village population. Age Ageing 1992;21(2): 121–8.

48. Martin MS, Sforza E, Roche F, et al, PROOF Study Group. Sleep breathing disorders and cognitive function in the elderly: an 8-year follow-up study. The Proof-Synapse cohort. Sleep 2015;38(2): 179–87.

49. Yesavage J, Bliwise D, Guilleminault C, et al. Preliminary communication: intellectual deficit and sleep-related respiratory disturbance in the elderly. Sleep 1985;8(1):30–3.

50. Alchanatis M, Zias N, Deligiorgis N, et al. Comparison of cognitive performance among different age groups in patients with obstructive sleep apnea. Sleep Breath 2008;12(1):17–24.

51. Crawford-Achour E, Dauphinot V, Saint Martin M, et al. Protective effect of long-term CPAP therapy on cognitive performance in elderly patients with severe OSA: the PROOF study. J Clin Sleep Med 2015; 11(5):519–24.

52. Ju G, Yoon I-Y, Lee SD, et al. Effects of sleep apnea syndrome on delayed memory and executive function in elderly adults. J Am Geriatr Soc 2012;60(6): 1099–103.

53. Berry DT, Phillips BA, Cook YR, et al. Geriatric sleep apnea syndrome: a preliminary description. J Gerontol 1990;45(5):M169–74.

54. Aloia MS, Ilniczky N, Di Dio P, et al. Neuropsychological changes and treatment compliance in older adults with sleep apnea. J Psychosom Res 2003; 54(1):71–6.

55. O'Hara R, Schröder CM, Kraemer HC, et al. Nocturnal sleep apnea/hypopnea is associated with lower memory performance in APOE ε4 carriers. Neurology 2005;65(4):642–4.

56. Osorio RS, Gumb T, Pirraglia E, et al. Sleep-disordered breathing advances cognitive decline in the elderly. Neurology 2015;84(19):1964–71.

57. Yaffe K, Laffan AM, Harrison SL, et al. Sleep-disordered breathing, hypoxia, and risk of mild cognitive impairment and dementia in older women. JAMA 2011;306(6):613–9.

58. Ancoli-Israel S, Ayalon L, Salzman C. Sleep in the elderly: normal variations and common sleep disorders. Harv Rev Psychiatry 2008;16(5):279–86.

59. Blackwell T, Yaffe K, Laffan A, et al. Associations between sleep-disordered breathing, nocturnal hypoxemia, and subsequent cognitive decline in older community-dwelling men: the Osteoporotic Fractures in Men Sleep Study. J Am Geriatr Soc 2015; 63(3):453–61.

60. Yaffe K, Falvey CM, Hoang T. Connections between sleep and cognition in older adults. Lancet Neurol 2014;13(10):1017–28.

61. Mathieu A, Mazza S, Décary A, et al. Effects of obstructive sleep apnea on cognitive function: a comparison between younger and older OSAS patients. Sleep Med 2008;9(2):112–20.

62. Boland LL, Shahar E, Iber C, et al. Measures of cognitive function in persons with varying degrees of sleep-disordered breathing: the Sleep Heart Health Study. J Sleep Res 2002;11(3):265–72.

63. Sforza E, Roche F, Thomas-Anterion C, et al. Cognitive function and sleep related breathing disorders

in a healthy elderly population: the SYNAPSE study. Sleep 2010;33(4):515–21.

64. Foley DJ, Masaki K, White L, et al. Sleep-disordered breathing and cognitive impairment in elderly Japanese-American men. Sleep 2003;26(5):596–9.

65. Portier F, Portmann A, Czernichow P, et al. Evaluation of home versus laboratory polysomnography in the diagnosis of sleep apnea syndrome. Am J Respir Crit Care Med 2000;162(3):814–8.

66. Beebe DW, Groesz L, Wells C, et al. The neuropsychological effects of obstructive sleep apnea: a meta-analysis of norm-referenced and case-controlled data. Sleep 2003;26(3):298–307.

67. Bucks RS, Olaithe M, Eastwood P. Neurocognitive function in obstructive sleep apnoea: a meta-review. Respirology 2013;18(1):61–70.

68. Ingram F, Henke KG, Levin HS, et al. Sleep apnea and vigilance performance in a community-dwelling older sample. Sleep 1994;17(3):248–52.

69. Kim SJ, Lee JH, Lee DY, et al. Neurocognitive dysfunction associated with sleep quality and sleep apnea in patients with mild cognitive impairment. Am J Geriatr Psychiatry 2011;19(4):374–81.

70. Dalmases M, Solé-Padullés C, Torres M, et al. Effect of CPAP on cognition, brain function, and structure among elderly patients with OSA: a randomized pilot study. Chest 2015;148(5):1214–23.

71. Kang S-H, Yoon I-Y, Lee SD, et al. Effects of continuous positive airway pressure treatment on cognitive functions in the Korean elderly with obstructive sleep apnea. Sleep Med Res 2016;7(1):10–5.

72. Cooke JR, Ancoli-Israel S, Liu L, et al. Continuous positive airway pressure deepens sleep in patients with Alzheimer's disease and obstructive sleep apnea. Sleep Med 2009;10(10):1101–6.

73. Russo-Magno P, O'Brien A, Panciera T, et al. Compliance with CPAP therapy in older men with obstructive sleep apnea. J Am Geriatr Soc 2001;49(9):1205–11.

74. Pilcher JJ, Band D, Odle-Dusseau HN, et al. Human performance under sustained operations and acute sleep deprivation conditions: toward a model of controlled attention. Aviat Space Environ Med 2007;78(Suppl 1):B15–24.

75. Harrison Y, Horne JA. The impact of sleep deprivation on decision making: a review. J Exp Psychol Appl 2000;6(3):236–49.

76. Bonnet MH, Arand DL. 24-hour metabolic rate in insomniacs and matched normal sleepers. Sleep 1995;18:581–8.

77. Richardson GS. Human physiological models of insomnia. Sleep Med 2007;8(Suppl 4):S9–14.

78. Dinges DF, Pack F, Williams K, et al. Cumulative sleepiness, mood disturbance and psychomotor vigilance performance decrements during a week of sleep restricted to 4-5 hours per night. Sleep 1997; 20(4):267–77.

79. Durmer JS, Dinges DF. Neurocognitive consequences of sleep deprivation. Semin Neurol 2005; 25(1):117–29.

80. Goel N, Rao H, Durmer JS, et al. Neurocognitive consequences of sleep deprivation. Semin Neurol 2009;29(4):320–39.

81. Boonstra TW, Stins JF, Daffertshofer A, et al. Effects of sleep deprivation on neural functioning: an integrative review. Cell Mol Life Sci 2007; 64(7–8):934–46.

Sleep and Nocturia in Older Adults

Camille P. Vaughan, MD, MS[a,b,]*, Donald L. Bliwise, PhD[c]

KEYWORDS

- Nocturia • Multicomponent • Insomnia • Aging

KEY POINTS

- Among older adults, nocturia is common, often occurs because of multiple chronic conditions or predisposing factors, and frequently coexists with sleep dysfunction.
- Multicomponent treatment emphasizing lifestyle and behavioral strategies should be considered as first-line therapy for older adults with nocturia.
- If lifestyle modification and behavioral treatment are not sufficient, multiple drug therapy options are available with modest ability to reduce nocturia episodes.
- Drug selection for management of nocturia may depend on the patient's underlying vulnerability to drug side effects with particular attention to the potential for adverse effects related to cognition and mobility/falls.
- In patients who are refractory to therapies that target the lower urinary tract, clinicians should consider formal evaluation of sleep dysfunction as a contributing cause of nocturia.

INTRODUCTION

Nocturia, defined as the complaint of awakening from sleep at night to void, occurs with increasing frequency as adults age. A recent systematic review reports nocturia incidence at a rate of 11.5% per year in persons more than 60 years of age, which is 4 times the rate for adults aged 40 to 50 years.[1] Previous studies suggest that nocturia is clinically significant and bothersome when it occurs at least twice nightly,[2] and that bother from nocturia is related to the magnitude of sleep disruption, particularly when returning to sleep after voiding is problematic.[3] At least 30% of older adults experience 2 or more episodes of nocturia per night.[4–6] Nocturia is associated with multiple negative health outcomes among older adults, including reduced quality of life, incident falls, sleep disturbance, and increased mortality.[7–14] Among older adults, nocturia typically occurs in the setting of multiple potential causes or risk factors, which lead to lower urinary tract dysfunction, increased urine production (either 24 hour or nighttime), sleep dysfunction, or a combination of these conditions.[15] This article considers the intersection of nocturia and sleep disturbance and recommends that a multicomponent approach is warranted to treat nocturia with comorbid sleep dysfunction in older adults.

MULTIFACTORIAL ASSESSMENT OF CONTRIBUTING CONDITIONS
Common Comorbid Conditions

Nocturia shares many features of a geriatric syndrome because it constitutes a combination of

Disclosure: Dr C.P. Vaughan's spouse is a full-time employee of Kimberly-Clark Corp. Dr D.L. Bliwise received fees from Ferring, Merck, and Vantia, and grants from the New England Research Institute.
[a] Birmingham/Atlanta Geriatric Research, Education, and Clinical Center, Atlanta VA Medical Center, Decatur, GA, USA; [b] Division of General Medicine and Geriatrics, Department of Medicine, Emory University, Atlanta, GA, USA; [c] Program in Sleep, Aging and Chronobiology, Department of Neurology, Emory University, 12 Executive Park Drive, Atlanta, GA 30329, USA
* Corresponding author. Wesley Woods Health Center, Emory University, 1841 Clifton Road, NorthEast, Room 533, Atlanta, GA 30329.
E-mail address: camille.vaughan@emory.edu

symptoms and signs that occur more often in older adults, leads to substantial morbidity, and occurs in the setting of multiple interacting and synergistic risk factors.[16] Nocturia may occur because of dysfunctional bladder storage, conditions associated with polyuria (ie, increased 24-hour urine production), nocturnal polyuria (ie, increased production of urine at night compared with daytime), or sleep disorders. However, in older adults, these conditions frequently coexist in the same individual and so the cause of nocturia is multifactorial. In addition, the relationship between sleep disruption and nocturia is bidirectional, which offers additional options for multicomponent treatment approaches.[17] The implication of this bidirectionality is that focusing treatment on sleep and sleep disorders may also reduce nocturnal voiding episodes. The initial evaluation of an older adult with nocturia and sleep disruption includes an assessment of contributing comorbid conditions. **Box 1** provides a summary of conditions to consider.

Medication Review

Providers should conduct a careful medication review to assess for drugs that increase nighttime urine production or polyuria. Strategies to modify medications include prescribing an alternative therapy or adjusting the timing of medications to reduce the impact on nighttime urine production. Commonly prescribed medications associated with nocturia include anticholinergic drugs, which cause dry mouth (which could lead to excessive fluid intake) and increase the risk of urinary retention. Calcium channel blockers may lead to salt diuresis by blocking proximal tubular secretion of sodium reabsorption or indirectly through promoting peripheral edema with overnight recirculation of dependent edema during recumbency. Diuretic therapy may be timed to avoid overnight diuresis and maximize the drug's effect during the daytime hours.

Physical Examination and Clinical Evaluation

The physical examination and additional assessments are targeted to determine contributing factors related to nocturia. If the patient has conditions that could contribute to volume overload (such as a history of congestive heart failure, liver or kidney disease), an evaluation of volume status is important. For men with symptoms consistent with overactive bladder, a rectal examination should be performed to assess for prostate enlargement. A rectal or vaginal examination also provides an opportunity to teach pelvic floor muscle contraction, which can be used as part of a behavioral therapy approach to nocturia.

Laboratory evaluation should include a urinalysis to assess for microscopic hematuria (defined as more than 5 red blood cells per high-powered field on 2 consecutive urinalyses without evidence of infection). If a urine culture is obtained, clinicians should consider that asymptomatic bacteriuria occurs in up to 20% of older women and 15% of older men.[18] Diagnosis of a urinary tract infection requires new patient-reported symptoms such as urinary storage symptoms, dysuria, or suprapubic pain, and culture of 1 bacterial species in a quantitative count of at least 10^5 colony-forming units (CFU) per milliliter in women and 10^3 CFU/mL in men.[19] Serum prostatic specific antigen (PSA) level is not routinely recommended in the assessment of men with lower urinary tract symptoms. The PSA test received a D recommendation (ie, harms outweigh benefits) from the United States Preventive Services Task Force. As of 2013, the American Urinary Association recommends shared decision making among men who are at average risk between the ages of 55 and 69 years in order to determine each man's values and preferences for PSA testing. Other testing may be indicated based on the patient's comorbid conditions,

---

Box 1
Conditions associated with nocturia among older adults

Conditions associated with detrusor hyperactivity

- Benign prostatic enlargement
- Overactive bladder
- Medication side effects
- Kidney or bladder stones

Conditions associated with polyuria or nocturnal polyuria

- Congestive heart failure on diuretic therapy
- Chronic kidney disease
- Diabetes: poorly controlled
- Lower extremity edema
- Excessive fluid intake
- Obstructive sleep apnea
- Diabetes insipidus

Conditions associated with sleep dysfunction

- Obstructive sleep apnea
- Rapid eye movement sleep behavior disorder
- Restless legs syndrome
- Periodic limb movement syndrome
- Shift work syndrome

such as hemoglobin A1c in diabetic patients if not checked within the previous 3 months to determine whether hyperglycemia is a contributor to nocturia.

A 24-hour frequency volume chart is key to determining the presence of nocturnal polyuria. Patients are instructed to measure urine output with each void for a 24-hour period. The time the patient goes to bed with the intention of going to sleep and the awakening time are recorded. The volume of urine that is produced overnight after sleep onset and including the first morning void are divided by the total 24-hour urine volume to determine the proportion of urine produced overnight. A proportion of nighttime urine production that is greater than one-third of the total urine production defines nocturnal polyuria in adults more than 65 years of age, which represents an age-adjusted value. Complex urodynamic evaluation is not routinely needed in the evaluation of nocturia. A postvoid residual (PVR) assessment by bladder ultrasonography can be useful, if available, to assess for urinary retention as a potential contributor.

Nocturia occurring at least 3 times nightly is associated with the presence of obstructive sleep apnea and referral for polysomnography should be considered, particularly if patients do not reach their treatment goals with initial treatment strategies.[20] Obstructive sleep apnea may lead to right heart strain and release of atrial natriuretic peptide, which leads to salt diuresis,[21] or to dysfunctional secretion of antidiuretic hormone, leading to increased urine production overnight.[22] Persons with untreated obstructive sleep apnea may experience awakenings because of hypoxemia overnight. During awakenings, bladder fullness may be perceived that otherwise would not have led to arousal.[23] In addition, it is estimated that up to half of older adults with nocturia experience insomnia.[24] Concurrent insomnia results in difficulty returning to sleep after an awakening and further exacerbates sleep disruption. Recent evidence suggests that interventions targeting poor sleep may also reduce nocturia episodes.[25] Thus, it is reasonable to assess for sleep dysfunction beyond obstructive sleep apnea as potential therapeutic targets to improve quality of life related to nocturia.

MULTICOMPONENT TREATMENT APPROACH
Lifestyle and Behavioral Treatment

Initial treatment strategies are informed by the identified contributors to nocturia. Multiple lifestyle and behavioral strategies may be considered and are listed in **Table 1**. For persons with lower extremity edema, daytime use of compression stockings prevents recirculation of dependent fluid accumulation while recumbent. For persons on chronic diuretic therapy, particularly loop diuretics, the timing of diuretic dosing should be reviewed to avoid diuresis overnight. Fluid intake may be reduced in the 2 to 3 hours before bedtime; however, some research suggests reducing fluid intake has limited impact on overnight urine production.[26] The type of fluid may be more important and so reducing the use of evening alcohol or caffeine is recommended in those experiencing bothersome nocturia.[27] Improving symptoms of dry mouth may aid in the avoidance of overnight fluid intake. Strategies to avoid xerostomia include reducing anticholinergic medications, avoiding alcohol-based mouthwash, or use of oral saliva replacement solution.

There is growing evidence for behavioral approaches to reduce nocturia episodes. Studies in men and women with nocturia suggest pelvic floor muscle exercise–based behavioral therapy that incorporates an urge suppression strategy is effective to treat nocturia.[28] Preliminary evidence suggests pelvic floor muscle exercise–based behavioral

Table 1
Lifestyle and behavioral strategies to treat nocturia

Strategy	Impact on Nocturia
Daytime compression stockings for peripheral edema	Prevent recirculation of dependent edema overnight
Restrict fluid intake 2–3 h before bedtime	May have modest impact to reduce urine output overnight
Manage xerostomia	Reduce fluid intake overnight
Pelvic floor muscle–based urge suppression	Suppress bladder muscle contractions and urge to void
Behavioral treatment of insomnia	Improve sleep and reduce the time to return to sleep after overnight awakenings

therapy has favorable effects compared with both α-blocker and bladder relaxant therapy in men and women.[29–31] Patients are instructed to practice pelvic floor muscle exercises daily (typically 45 exercises per day, which may be performed while lying, sitting, or standing at any time of day) in order to strengthen the pelvic floor and automate the pelvic floor muscle contraction technique. The urge suppression strategy involves remaining still on awakening with the urge to void at night; squeezing the pelvic floor muscles rapidly several times in a row, which inhibits bladder muscle contraction; and using a mindfulness technique to concentrate on suppressing the urge. Once the urge subsides, patients are instructed to try to return to sleep. If they are unable to return to sleep because of the need to void, they are instructed to use the urge suppression strategy before arising from bed in order to avoid being in the midst of urgency when walking to the toilet. Behavioral therapy targeting nocturia also seems to improve some aspects of sleep, such as reducing wakefulness after sleep onset.[29,32] One study suggests that increasing the duration of sleep before the first awakening to void may improve overall sleep quality.[33] In addition to pelvic floor muscle exercise–based behavioral therapy, brief behavioral therapy for insomnia has shown preliminary impact to reduce nocturia,[25] and behavioral therapy for nocturia has a favorable impact on sleep.[29,32] Future research should evaluate combination behavioral therapy for insomnia and behavioral interventions for nocturia.

For men with mobility impairment, a bedside urinal to prevent the need to walk to the bathroom at night should be considered. A bedside commode is another option in men or women with mobility impairment. Containment strategies include absorptive undergarments and bed pads to reduce leakage of urine. In men, a condom catheter may be considered, although external catheters increase the risk of urinary tract infection compared with absorptive undergarments. A barrier cream at night may prevent the development of skin irritation from wetness, which could be another source of awakening overnight.

Pharmacologic Treatment

Drug therapies focused on the lower urinary tract typically result in modest nocturia reductions (Table 2).[30,31,34] α-Blockers could be considered in men who have evidence of prostate enlargement and other symptoms of overactive bladder, such as urgency and frequency. Although the risk of orthostatic hypotension is decreased with selective α1-adrenergic receptor antagonists, which have greater affinity for the receptors in the lower urinary tract (α_{1a} subtype; ie, tamsulosin, silodosin), significant orthostasis may still occur in up to 1 in 12 men on these agents.[35] On physical examination, if the patient's blood pressure is low normal (<110/70 mm Hg) and the patient is already taking antihypertensive therapy, it may be judicious to hold antihypertensive therapy during the initiation of even a prostate-selective α-antagonist. Patients should be instructed about the potential for dizziness or light-headedness and to discontinue therapy if these symptoms become prominent. In men with an enlarged prostate on examination or a PSA level greater than 1.5 ng/mL, 5α-reductase inhibitors may be useful. Although there is an overall reduced risk of prostate cancer, there is an increased risk of moderate-grade to high-grade prostate cancer.[36] In 2 studies, a 5α-reductase inhibitor alone had modest effect to reduce nocturia compared with placebo; however, in combination with an α-blocker, the reduction was more significant.[34,37] Daily type 5 phosphodiesterase inhibitors (PDE5i) are another option for men with lower urinary tract symptoms related to prostate enlargement who are not candidates for α-blocker therapy or as add-on therapy to α-blockers selective for the prostatic α1a receptor (tadalafil is the only PDE5i with US Food and Drug Administration [FDA] approval). The effect of tadalafil to reduce nocturia frequency, although statistically significant compared with placebo, is not considered clinically significant.[38] Phosphodiesterase inhibitors may be associated with increased risk of hypotension.[36] In addition, melatonin is another option for treatment of nocturia among men with prostate enlargement.[39] Melatonin may not affect the prostate directly; however, sleep dysfunction commonly occurs in the setting of nocturia and melatonin has been shown in some studies to be a treatment of insomnia in older adults. Melatonin is typically dosed between 3 and 10 mg up to 2 hours before bedtime.

Bladder relaxant therapy may be appropriate in those who do not have an increased postvoid residual at baseline.[40] Antimuscarinic bladder relaxants reduce the action of acetylcholine to influence detrusor muscle contraction by competitively binding muscarinic receptors but also may reduce afferent sensory signaling from bladder C-fibers and Aδ-fibers.[41] Because antimuscarinic agents vary in their affinity for the bladder muscarinic receptor subtypes (M2 and M3) and in their likelihood to cross the blood-brain barrier, there is additional concern about the potential for cognitive side effects.[42,43] Few studies have been designed to specifically evaluate the cognitive impact of antimuscarinic medications among older adults. One randomized controlled trial in healthy older adults

Table 2
Drug therapy related to lower urinary tract function to treat nocturia

Drugs	Dosages	Mechanisms of Action	Potential Adverse Effects
Bladder relaxants	In general, reduced dosages for renal and hepatic impairment	Increase bladder capacity; diminish involuntary bladder contractions	—
Darifenacin (Enablex)	7.5–15 mg qd	—	Anticholinergic, lower dose if reduced hepatic function
Fesoterodine (Toviaz)	4–8 mg qd	—	Anticholinergic
Mirabegron (Myrbetriq)	25–50 mg qd	—	Beta3-agonist, maximum 25 mg/d with CrCl 15–29 mL/min, reduced hepatic function; hypertension, tachycardia
Oxybutynin (Ditropan, immediate release, available as generic)	2.5–5.0 mg tid	—	Anticholinergic (dry mouth, blurry vision, increased intraocular pressure, delirium, constipation)
Oxybutynin (extended release) (Ditropan XL)	5–30 mg qd (most often 10 mg qd)	—	As above, but with less dry mouth
Patch (Oxytrol)	3.9 mg qd	Patch applied twice weekly	As above, but with less dry mouth, available over the counter
Oxybutynin gel (Gelnique)	3% pump or 10% gel packet	One application daily	As above, but with less dry mouth
Solifenacin (Vesicare)	5–10 mg qd	—	Anticholinergic, lower for severe renal impairment or reduced hepatic function
Tolterodine (Detrol)	1–2 mg bid	—	Anticholinergic, lower dose for severe renal impairment or reduced hepatic function
Tolterodine (Detrol LA)	4 mg qd	—	As above, but with less dry mouth
Trospium chloride (Sanctura)	20 mg bid	—	Anticholinergic, 20 mg once daily qhs with CrCl <30 mL/min or in patients >75 y old
Trospium chloride (Sanctura XR)	60 mg qam	—	Avoid in severe renal impairment or reduced hepatic function
α-Adrenergic Antagonist			
Doxazosin (available as generic, or Cardura)	1–8 mg qhs (higher dose typically necessary for urinary symptoms associated with prostatic enlargement)	Relax smooth muscle of urethra and prostatic capsule	Postural hypotension, dizziness, reduces blood pressure

(continued on next page)

Table 2
(continued)

Drugs	Dosages	Mechanisms of Action	Potential Adverse Effects
Terazosin (available as generic, or Hytrin)	1–20 mg qhs (at least 10 mg dose typically necessary for urinary symptoms associated with prostatic enlargement)	—	Same as above
Prazosin (Minipress)	1–2 mg bid	—	Same as above
Alfuzosin (Uroxatral)	10 mg qhs	—	Less effect on blood pressure
Silodosin (Rapaflo)	8 mg qd	—	Less effect on blood pressure; CrCl 30–50 mL/min use 4 mg qd
Tamsulosin (Flomax)	0.4–0.8 mg qd	—	Less effect on blood pressure (when used at 0.8-mg dose, greater blood pressure effects)
Phosphodiesterase Inhibitor			
Tadalafil	5 mg daily	Inhibits PDE type 5, enhancing effects of nitric oxide-activated increases in cGMP	Orthostatic hypotension, flushing, headache (contraindicated with terazosin/doxazosin/prazosin)
Other phosphodiesterase inhibitors given daily may be effective	—	—	—
5α-reductase inhibitor	—	Inhibits type II 5αreductase, interfering with conversion of testosterone to 5α-dihydrotestosterone	—
Finasteride	5 mg daily	—	Sexual dysfunction, gynecomastia, decreased overall risk of prostate cancer with increased risk of high-grade prostate cancer
Dutasteride	0.5 mg daily	Inhibits type I and II 5α-reductase, inhibiting conversion of testosterone to dihydrotestosterone	Sexual dysfunction, decreased overall risk of prostate cancer with increased risk of high-grade prostate cancer

Abbreviations: bid, twice a day; cGMP, cyclic guanosine monophosphate; CrCl, creatinine clearance; PDE, phosphodiesterase; qam, every morning; qd, every day; qhs, at night; tid, 3 times a day.

Data from American Geriatrics Society and Talebreza S, editor. Geriatrics Evaluation & Management Tools. New York: American Geriatrics Society; 2016. Available at: https://geriatricscareonline.org/toc/geriatrics-evaluation-management-tools/B007.

more than 60 years of age (range, 60–83 years) with no baseline cognitive impairment showed that a dosage of oxybutynin extended release greater than 10 mg daily was associated with decline in cognitive function compared with placebo or darifenacin dosed at 7.5 mg or 15 mg daily.[44] Although further research studies regarding effects on cognition are needed, all antimuscarinic drugs are associated with the side effects of dry mouth and constipation. Combination therapy with an α-blocker and antimuscarinic drug may be effective to reduce nocturia, although studies of combined therapy specifically for nocturia are limited.[45] Beta3-agonists are another class of bladder relaxant medications that lead to bladder smooth muscle relaxation when the beta3-receptor is stimulated. At present, there is 1 FDA-approved medication in this class for lower urinary tract symptoms (mirabegron). Beta3-agonists avoid the anticholinergic side effects associated with antimuscarinic agents. However, mirabegron is not recommended in persons with uncontrolled hypertension or in those with significant arrhythmias. Additional evidence is needed to assess the impact of mirabegron specifically for nocturia. A study comparing mirabegron with antimuscarinic drug therapy showed similar effects to reduce nocturia (a reduction of 0.4 episodes per night on average)[46]; however, another study comparing mirabegron with both antimuscarinic drug therapy and placebo showed no significantly different nocturia reduction between mirabegron and placebo.[47]

It is unclear whether nocturnal polyuria, as determined by measures recorded in a 24-hour frequency volume chart, modifies the response to behavioral or drug therapy targeting lower urinary tract function. One study suggested that persons with nocturnal polyuria did not respond to bladder relaxant therapy for nocturia.[40] Another recent study suggests that the presence of nocturnal polyuria did not affect the response to behavioral or combination behavioral and α-blocker treatment of nocturia.[29] Although achieving antidiuresis via administration of a synthetic vasopressin analogue (desmopressin) has been a successful treatment of enuresis in children, concerns exist about the use of such therapy to treat nocturnal polyuria in older adults because of the risk of symptomatic hyponatremia. Desmopressin is included among a list of medications considered potentially inappropriate among older adults as determined by the Beers Criteria as applied by an expert consensus panel convened by the American Geriatrics Society in 2015.[48] The safety of recent ultralow-dose formulations (ie, microgram vs milligram) remains to be seen, although recent approvals of such formulations outside the United States should soon yield

relevant data for this issue. In frail older adults with urinary incontinence,[49] or elderly adults with certain comorbidities such as congestive heart failure with concomitant diuretic use, any usage of desmopressin as a treatment of nocturia is ill-advised.

In women who have evidence of atrophic vaginitis on examination, low-dose topical estrogen can reduce urgency, frequency, and urinary incontinence.[50] If these symptoms are contributing to nighttime awakenings and nocturia episodes, it may be reasonable to consider treatment. Although systemic absorption is minimal when estrogen cream is used in low doses (0.5 g applied 3 times a week), topical estrogen likely should not be used in women who have a personal history of breast cancer.[51] Once the vaginal epithelium is restored, the dosing frequency should be decreased to the minimum needed to prevent recurrent symptoms. Among women who have a contraindication to topical estrogen, personal lubricants may be an alternative to reduce skin irritation.

Minimally Invasive and Surgical Treatment

Minimally invasive and surgical procedures have been studied in the context of persons with overactive bladder syndrome and incontinence who have failed lifestyle, behavioral, and drug therapies; however, there is less evidence specifically for the treatment of nocturia. It is unclear exactly how neuromodulation affects overactive bladder syndrome, but it is hypothesized that stimulation of afferent fibers from the bladder leads to central inhibition of bladder motor neurons, resulting in less detrusor hyperactivity.[52] Percutaneous tibial nerve stimulation is minimally invasive and requires weekly visits to the clinic for up to 12 weeks followed by an individualized tapering protocol for long-term therapy, which could be burdensome. A 36-month follow-up study of percutaneous tibial nerve stimulation suggests a sustained reduction on average of 0.5 episodes per night.[53] Another form of modulation is sacral neuromodulation with an implanted stimulator device. Data specific to nighttime voiding episodes have not been reported in long-term studies of sacral neuromodulation.[54]

The use of cystoscopic injection of Botulinum toxin for overactive bladder received approval in the United States with a recommended total intravesical dosage of 200 units. Results from a multisite study of persons with refractory overactive bladder receiving cystoscopic injections totaling 100 units of onabotulinumtoxinA revealed an average nocturia reduction of 0.5 episodes per night at 12 weeks postinjection.[55] Urinary retention requiring intermittent catheterization for up to 3 months can occur and is more likely if an increased PVR is present before the injection. Repeat injections are typically required within 6 to 12 months.

Concomitant prostate enlargement is common in older men with nocturia. There are a variety of less invasive prostate reduction procedures, including needle or microwave thermotherapy, that may be considered in men who are not candidates for laser ablation or transurethral resection of the prostate (TURP). The ability of TURP to improve nocturia is less well studied. One study suggests that reduction in nocturia frequency associated with TURP does not correlate with improvements in sleep quality.[56] Surgical interventions for women that target stress incontinence do not generally improve lower urinary tract symptoms associated with overactive bladder syndrome.

SUMMARY

Nocturia is common among older adults and frequently coexists with sleep dysfunction and other comorbid chronic conditions. A multicomponent treatment approach that emphasizes lifestyle and behavioral strategies should be considered as first-line treatment of older adults. Multiple drug therapy options are available with modest impact to reduce nocturia episodes. Drug selection may depend on the patient's underlying vulnerability to drug side effects with particular attention to the potential for adverse effects related to cognition, mobility, and falls. In patients who are refractory to therapies that target the lower urinary tract, clinicians should consider formal evaluation for sleep dysfunction as a contributing cause.

REFERENCES

1. Pesonen JS, Cartwright R, Mangera A, et al. Incidence and remission of nocturia: a systematic review and meta-analysis. Eur Urol 2016;70(2): 372–81.
2. Tikkinen KAO, Johnson TM II, Tammela TLJ, et al. Nocturia frequency, bother, and quality of life: how often is too often? A population-based study in Finland. Eur Urol 2010;57(3):488–98.
3. Vaughan CP, Eisenstein R, Bliwise DL, et al. Self-rated sleep characteristics and bother from nocturia. Int J Clin Pract 2012;66(4):369–73.
4. Burgio KL, Johnson Ii TM, Goode PS, et al. Prevalence and correlates of nocturia in community-dwelling older adults. J Am Geriatr Soc 2010;58(5): 861–6.
5. Markland AD, Vaughan CP, Johnson Ii TM, et al. Prevalence of nocturia in United States men: results from the National Health and Nutrition Examination Survey. J Urol 2011;185(3):998–1002.
6. Coyne KS, Zhou Z, Bhattacharyya SK, et al. The prevalence of nocturia and its effect on health-related quality of life and sleep in a community sample in the USA. BJU Int 2003;92(9):948–54.
7. Bliwise DL, Rosen RC, Baum N. Impact of nocturia on sleep and quality of life: a brief, selected review for the International Consultation on Incontinence Research Society (ICI-RS) nocturia think tank. Neurourol Urodyn 2014;33(S1):S15–8.
8. Yu H-J, Chen F-Y, Huang P-C, et al. Impact of nocturia on symptom-specific quality of life among community-dwelling adults aged 40 years and older. Urology 2006;67(4):713–8.
9. Vaughan CP, Brown CJ, Goode PS, et al. The association of nocturia with incident falls in an elderly community-dwelling cohort. Int J Clin Pract 2010; 64(5):577–83.
10. Parthasarathy S, Fitzgerald M, Goodwin JL, et al. Nocturia, sleep-disordered breathing, and cardiovascular morbidity in a community-based cohort. PLoS One 2012;7(2):e30969.
11. Bliwise DL, Foley DJ, Vitiello MV, et al. Nocturia and disturbed sleep in the elderly. Sleep Med 2009; 10(5):540–8.
12. Kupelian V, Fitzgerald MP, Kaplan SA, et al. Association of nocturia and mortality: results from the Third National Health and Nutrition Examination Survey. J Urol 2011;185(2):571–7.
13. Endeshaw YW, Schwartz AV, Stone KL, et al. Nocturia, insomnia symptoms, and mortality among older men: the health, aging and body composition study. J Clin Sleep Med 2016;12:789–96.
14. Vaughan CP, Fung CH, Huang AJ, et al. Differences in the association of nocturia and functional outcomes of sleep by age and gender: a cross-sectional, population-based study. Clin Ther 2016; 38(11):2386–93.e1.
15. Weiss JP, Juul KV, Wein A. Management of nocturia: the role of antidiuretic pharmacotherapy. Neurourol Urodyn 2014;33:S19–24.
16. Inouye SK, Studenski S, Tinetti ME, et al. Geriatric syndromes: clinical, research, and policy implications of a core geriatric concept. J Am Geriatr Soc 2007;55(5):780–91.
17. Araujo AB, Yaggi HK, Yang M, et al. Sleep-related problems and urologic symptoms: testing the hypothesis of bi-directionality in a longitudinal, population-based study. J Urol 2014;191(1):100–6.
18. Nicolle LE. Asymptomatic bacteriuria: when to screen and when to treat. Infect Dis Clin North Am 2003;17(2):367–94.
19. Nicolle LE. Urinary tract infections in the elderly. Clin Geriatr Med 2009;25(3):423–36.

20. Endeshaw YW, Johnson TM, Kutner MH, et al. Sleep-disordered breathing and nocturia in older adults. J Am Geriatr Soc 2004;52(6):957–60.

21. Krieger J, Laks L, Wilcox I, et al. Atrial natriuretic peptide release during sleep in patients with obstructive sleep apnoea before and during treatment with nasal continuous positive airway pressure. Clin Sci 1989;77:407–11.

22. Ozben S, Guvenc TS, Huseyinoglu N, et al. Low serum copeptin levels in patients with obstructive sleep apnea. Sleep Breath 2013;17(4):1187–92.

23. Pressman MR, Figueroa WG, Kendrick-Mohamed J, et al. Nocturia: a rarely recognized symptom of sleep apnea and other occult sleep disorders. Arch Intern Med 1996;156(5):545–50.

24. Zeitzer JM, Bliwise DL, Hernandez BA, et al. Nocturia compounds nocturnal wakefulness in older individuals with insomnia. J Clin Sleep Med 2013;9(3):259–62.

25. Tyagi S, Resnick NM, Perera S, et al. Behavioral treatment of insomnia: also effective for nocturia. J Am Geriatr Soc 2014;62(1):54–60.

26. Johnson TM, Sattin RW, Parmelee P, et al. Evaluating potentially modifiable risk factors for prevalent and incident nocturia in older adults. J Am Geriatr Soc 2005;53(6):1011–6.

27. Soda T, Masui K, Okuno H, et al. Efficacy of nondrug lifestyle measures for the treatment of nocturia. J Urol 2010;184(3):1000–4.

28. Yap TL, Brown C, Cromwell DA, et al. The impact of self-management of lower urinary tract symptoms on frequency-volume chart measures. BJU Int 2009;104(8):1104–8.

29. Johnson TM II, Vaughan CP, Goode PS, et al. Pilot results from a randomized trial in men comparing alpha-adrenergic antagonist versus behavior and exercise for nocturia and sleep. Clin Ther 2016;38(11):2394–406.e3.

30. Johnson TM, Markland AD, Goode PS, et al. Efficacy of adding behavioural treatment or antimuscarinic drug therapy to α-blocker therapy in men with nocturia. BJU Int 2013;112(1):100–8.

31. Johnson TM, Burgio KL, Redden DT, et al. Effects of behavioral and drug therapy on nocturia in older incontinent women. J Am Geriatr Soc 2005;53(5):846–50.

32. Vaughan CP, Endeshaw Y, Nagamia Z, et al. A multicomponent behavioural and drug intervention for nocturia in elderly men: rationale and pilot results. BJU Int 2009;104(1):69–74.

33. Bliwise DL, Holm-Larsen T, Goble S, et al. Short time to first void is associated with lower whole-night sleep quality in nocturia patients. J Clin Sleep Med 2015;11(1):53–5.

34. Johnson TM II, Burrows PK, Kusek JW, et al. The effect of doxazosin, finasteride and combination therapy on nocturia in men with benign prostatic hyperplasia. J Urol 2007;178(5):2045–51.

35. Fine SR, Ginsberg P. Alpha-adrenergic receptor antagonists in older patients with benign prostatic hyperplasia: issues and potential complications. J Am Osteopath Assoc 2008;108(7):333–7.

36. Sarma AV, Wei JT. Benign prostatic hyperplasia and lower urinary tract symptoms. N Engl J Med 2012;367(3):248–57.

37. Johnson TM II, Jones K, Williford WO, et al. Changes in nocturia from medical treatment of benign prostatic hyperplasia: secondary analysis of the Department of Veterans Affairs Cooperative Study Trial. J Urol 2003;170(1):145–8.

38. Oelke M, Weiss JP, Mamoulakis C, et al. Effects of tadalafil on nighttime voiding (nocturia) in men with lower urinary tract symptoms suggestive of benign prostatic hyperplasia: a post hoc analysis of pooled data from four randomized, placebo-controlled clinical studies. World J Urol 2014;32(5):1127–32.

39. Drake MJ, Mills IW, Noble JG. Melatonin pharmacotherapy for nocturia in men with benign prostatic enlargement. J Urol 2004;171(3):1199–202.

40. Brubaker L, FitzGerald MP. Nocturnal polyuria and nocturia relief in patients treated with solifenacin for overactive bladder symptoms. Int Urogynecol J 2007;18(7):737–41.

41. Andersson K-E. Antimuscarinic mechanisms and the overactive detrusor: an update. Eur Urol 2011;59(3):377–86.

42. Kay GG, Abou-Donia MB, Messer WS, et al. Antimuscarinic drugs for overactive bladder and their potential effects on cognitive function in older patients. J Am Geriatr Soc 2005;53(12):2195–201.

43. Andersson K-E, Chapple CR, Cardozo L, et al. Pharmacological treatment of overactive bladder: report from the International Consultation on Incontinence. Curr Opin Urol 2009;19(4):380–94.

44. Kay G, Crook T, Rekeda L, et al. Differential effects of the antimuscarinic agents darifenacin and oxybutynin ER on memory in older subjects. Eur Urol 2006;50(2):317–26.

45. Kaplan SA, Roehrborn CG, Rovner ES, et al. Tolterodine and tamsulosin for treatment of men with lower urinary tract symptoms and overactive bladder: a randomized controlled trial. JAMA 2006;296(19):2319–28.

46. Chapple CR, Kaplan SA, Mitcheson D, et al. Randomized double-blind, active-controlled phase 3 study to assess 12-month safety and efficacy of mirabegron, a β3-adrenoceptor agonist, in overactive bladder. Eur Urol 2013;63(2):296–305.

47. Kuo H-C, Lee K-S, Na Y, et al. Results of a randomized, double-blind, parallel-group, placebo- and active-controlled, multicenter study of mirabegron, a β3-adrenoceptor agonist, in patients with

overactive bladder in Asia. Neurourol Urodyn 2015;34(7):685–92.

48. American Geriatrics Society 2015 Beers Criteria Update Expert Panel. American Geriatrics Society 2015 updated Beers criteria for potentially inappropriate medication use in older adults. J Am Geriatr Soc 2015;63(11):2227–46.

49. Thüroff JW, Abrams P, Andersson K-E, et al. EAU guidelines on urinary incontinence. Eur Urol 2011; 59(3):387–400.

50. Cardozo L, Bachmann G, McClish D, et al. Meta-analysis of estrogen therapy in the management of urogenital atrophy in postmenopausal women: second report of the Hormones and Urogenital Therapy Committee. Obstet Gynecol 1998;92(Supplement): 722–7.

51. Ponzone R, Biglia N, Jacomuzzi ME, et al. Vaginal oestrogen therapy after breast cancer: is it safe? Eur J Cancer 2005;41(17):2673–81.

52. Kabay SC, Kabay S, Yucel M, et al. Acute urodynamic effects of percutaneous posterior tibial nerve stimulation on neurogenic detrusor overactivity in patients with Parkinson's disease. Neurourol Urodyn 2009;28(1):62–7.

53. Peters KM, Carrico DJ, Wooldridge LS, et al. Percutaneous tibial nerve stimulation for the long-term treatment of overactive bladder: 3-year results of the STEP study. J Urol 2013;189(6):2194–201.

54. Noblett K, Siegel S, Mangel J, et al. Results of a prospective, multicenter study evaluating quality of life, safety, and efficacy of sacral neuromodulation at twelve months in subjects with symptoms of overactive bladder. Neurourol Urodyn 2016;35(2):246–51.

55. Chapple C, Sievert K-D, MacDiarmid S, et al. OnabotulinumtoxinA 100 U significantly improves all idiopathic overactive bladder symptoms and quality of life in patients with overactive bladder and urinary incontinence: a randomised, double-blind, placebo-controlled trial. Eur Urol 2013;64(2):249–56.

56. Wada N, Numata A, Hou K, et al. Nocturia and sleep quality after transurethral resection of the prostate. Int J Urol 2014;21(1):81–5.

Sleep and Long-Term Care

Lichuan Ye, PhD, RN[a], Kathy C. Richards, PhD, RN[b],*

KEYWORDS

- Sleep disturbance • Long-term care • Nursing homes • Older adults

KEY POINTS

- Long-term care (LTC) involves a range of support and services for people with chronic illness and disabilities who can not perform activities of daily living independently.
- Poor sleep increases the risk of LTC placement, and sleep disturbance is extremely common among LTC residents.
- The identification and management of sleep disturbance in LTC residents is a vital, but perhaps underappreciated, aspect of offering high-quality care for this already compromised population.
- This review describes the nature and consequences of sleep disturbances in LTC, clinical assessment and management of sleep disturbances in LTC, and implications for future research and clinical practice.

Long-term care (LTC) involves a range of support and services for people with chronic illness and disabilities who can not perform activities of daily living independently. It is expected that approximately 70% of adults older than 65 years of age will use some form of LTC.[1] For the purpose of this review, only studies of facility-based LTC settings are included, such as nursing homes, assisted living facilities, and continuing care retirement communities. Poor sleep increases the risk of LTC placement,[2] and sleep disturbance is extremely common among LTC residents.[3] The identification and management of sleep disturbance in LTC residents is a vital, but perhaps underappreciated, aspect of offering high-quality care for this already compromised population.[4] This review describes the nature and consequences of sleep disturbances in LTC, the clinical assessment and management of sleep disturbances in LTC, and the implications for future research and clinical practice.

POOR SLEEP AND THE RISK OF LONG-TERM CARE PLACEMENT

Spira and colleagues[2] prospectively examined whether poor sleep increased the risk of institutionalization in a large cohort of community-dwelling older women. They found that greater sleep fragmentation measured by wrist actigraphy substantially increased the likelihood of LTC placement after 5 years.[2]

Poor sleep may contribute to the increased risk of LTC placement for a variety of reasons. One explanation is that poor sleep leads to cognitive impairment. A metaanalysis of 77 studies among regional or national representative samples of older adults identified cognitive impairment as a key predictor of nursing home placement.[5] Recent prospective cohort studies, using both objective and subjective measures of sleep quality, offered strong evidence that poor sleep led to cognitive decline in older adults.[6,7] It is also possible that

Disclosure Statement: Dr K.C. Richards has no financial conflicts of interest. She has funding from the National Institutes of Health (R01AG051588 and R01AG054435) and has received CPAP units from Philips Respironics for a study on the effect of CPAP on persons with mild cognitive impairment. Dr L. Ye has no relevant conflict of interest. She received research funding from the National Institutes of Health and Agency for Healthcare Research and Quality (R21 HS24330).
a Bouvé College of Health Sciences School of Nursing, Northeastern University, Boston, MA 02115, USA; b The University of Texas at Austin, School of Nursing, 1710 Red River, Austin, TX 78701, USA
* Corresponding author.
E-mail address: kricha@utexas.edu

Sleep Med Clin 13 (2018) 117–125
https://doi.org/10.1016/j.jsmc.2017.09.011
1556-407X/18/© 2017 Elsevier Inc. All rights reserved.

frequent nocturnal awakenings increase caregiver burden and stress, which prompts the institutionalization of older adults receiving care at home.[8] However, one could argue that poor sleep in care recipients may not necessarily be linked to disturbed sleep in caregivers.[9] Some other explanations of how poor sleep increases the risk of LTC placement include sleep loss linked to chronic inflammation leading to functional impairment and declining health.[10,11] Poor sleep may also be a side effect of prescribed medications, or it can be a sign of other comorbidities known to increase risk for institutionalization among older adults, such as depression.

Future research is necessary to discover the mechanisms linking sleep disturbance to the increased risk for LTC placement, and to evaluate if sleep promotion strategies could decrease the risk of institutionalization. As an attempt to prevent LTC placement, clinicians working with older adults should assess sleep on a regular basis, closely monitor individuals with highly fragmented or insufficient sleep, and provide nonpharmacologic strategies for improving sleep whenever possible.

SLEEP DISTURBANCE IN LONG-TERM CARE

Although common in older adults, sleep disturbances are even more prevalent and more severe in institutionalized older adults.[12] Compared with community-dwelling older adults, LTC residents with and without dementia showed significantly lower sleep efficiency, longer awake time, and more sleep fragmentation throughout the night as measured by actigraphy.[13] In a study of 334 nursing home residents, 72.1% of the residents were classified as poor sleepers, and 49.6% were taking hypnotic medications.[3] Poor sleep in LTC residents is common across countries and cultures. In a recent study of more than 4000 elderly nursing home residents from Israel and 7 European countries, the overall prevalence of insomnia was 24% (ranging from 13% to >30%). In this study, insomnia was defined by the presence of symptoms of difficulty falling asleep or staying asleep, waking up too early, restlessness, or nonrestful sleep at any time.[14] Sleep disturbances are not only common, but they can also be persistent for up to 6 to 12 months, as reported in various LTC settings.[15,16] The persistence of sleep disturbance may have profound impact on LTC residents.

CONSEQUENCES OF SLEEP DISTURBANCE IN LONG-TERM CARE

A large body of evidence exists supporting the negative consequences of poor sleep or sleep disturbance in general. For example, poor sleep is associated with worse physical function, including gait speed, in older adults.[17] Sleep disturbance can adversely affect neuronal health, as supported by the observation that changes in sleep pattern increase the risk for dementia.[18] Studies in LTC residents have linked sleep disturbance to decreased functional status,[3] less functional recovery with rehabilitation,[19] social disengagement,[20] greater risk of falls,[21] frailty,[22] agitation,[23] and higher mortality.[24]

CLINICAL ASSESSMENT OF SLEEP DISTURBANCE IN LONG-TERM CARE

The diagnosis of sleep disturbance in residents of LTC is based on an in-depth clinical history from residents (if able), family members, and LTC staff; observations of daytime and nighttime sleep; and a physical examination. If indicated, polysomnography, sleep logs, actigraphy, questionnaires such as the Pittsburg Sleep Quality Index,[25] the Behavioral Indicators Test—Restless Legs,[26] STOP-Bang to screen for obstructive sleep apnea (OSA),[27] and other diagnostics may be required. A referral to a sleep specialist may be indicated when a sleep disorder is suspected.[28] Before initiating treatment, characteristics and causes of sleep disturbances must be carefully investigated, and a diagnosis established.[29] Careful evaluation can help clinicians to avoid inappropriate treatments or missing important symptoms related to poor sleep quality.

FACTORS THAT CONTRIBUTE TO SLEEP DISTURBANCE IN LONG-TERM CARE

Sleep disturbance in LTC residents is likely to result from a variety of individual and environmental factors,[30] including age-related changes in sleep architecture, environmental noise, nocturnal care practices, physical inactivity, social disengagement, depression, dementia, sleep disorders, and polypharmacy.[31] Understanding these factors will inform the development of strategies to improve sleep for LTC residents. **Box 1** summarizes the factors that contribute to sleep disturbance in LTC.

Age-Related Factors

Older age independently predicts the existence of sleep disturbance in LTC residents.[14] Sleep in older adults is characterized by frequent arousals, decreased deep sleep, and advanced sleep phase with the tendency to fall asleep earlier in the evening and wake up earlier in the morning.[32] Although poor sleep should not be considered as a normal part of aging, age-related changes in

Box 1
Factors that contribute to sleep disturbance in long-term care

Age-related factors
- Changes in sleep architecture
- Advanced sleep phase
- Weakening of circadian entertainment
- Visual impairment

Environmental factors
- Daytime limited exposure to bright light
- Nighttime environmental noise, light, and unpleasant temperature
- Room sharing
- Nocturnal care activities and facility routines

Behavioral factors
- Reduced daytime physical activity
- Reduced social activities and social disengagement
- Excessive daytime napping

Medical and psychiatric factors
- Incontinence and nocturia
- Symptoms such as pain and dyspnea
- Dementia or cognitive impairment
- Depression
- Sleep disorders such as insomnia, obstructive sleep apnea, and restless legs syndrome
- Side effects of medications

sleep architecture and weakening of circadian entertainment may contribute to the sleep disturbance commonly seen in LTC residents.

Environmental Factors

Sleep in LTC can be interrupted by environmental factors such as noise, lighting, room temperature, room sharing, and nocturnal care activities. With residents seldom being taken outdoors, limited exposure to bright light during the day significantly contributes to circadian deregulation.[33] Environmental noise and incontinence care practices at night are responsible for a substantial amount of sleep disruption among LTC residents.[34] A recent national survey revealed that health care providers' knowledge of sleep was limited, and there was a general lack of awareness regarding sleep disturbance for patients with dementia.[35] This limited knowledge and lack of awareness from professionals may lead to care activities

scheduled for the convenience of the staff even when they interfere with the residents' sleep.

Behavioral Factors

LTC residents tend to spend extended time in bed, are physically inactive, and are less engaged in social activities during the daytime.[36] Reduced daytime physical and social activities in LTC residents significantly contribute to their circadian rhythm abnormalities resulting in excessive daytime sleepiness and disturbed nighttime sleep.[36] Daytime napping is common among older LTC residents.[37] Although there is considerable controversy about the health-related consequences of napping among older adults, excessive daytime napping may lead to decreased nocturnal sleep and alter the sleep–wake cycle. Emotional distress, isolation, loneliness, and the process of relocation to an LTC facility often lead to social disengagement and contribute to nocturnal sleep disturbances.[31]

Medical and Psychiatric Factors

Sleep complaints in older adults are often secondary to comorbidities.[38] The majority of LTC residents suffer from multiple chronic conditions that contribute to sleep disruptions, such as depression, dementia, chronic pain, nocturia, heart failure, and pulmonary diseases. For example, more than one-half of LTC residents have some form of dementia or cognitive impairment,[39] which may increase sleep fragmentation and excessive daytime sleepiness.[40]

Nearly all residents take multiple medications to manage medical and psychiatric conditions.[41] It is highly likely that some medications impact nighttime sleep and/or daytime alertness. Medications like diuretics or sympathomimetics can be particularly problematic when taken near bedtime.

Sleep disorders are common but may be underdiagnosed and undertreated among LTC residents. At least 40% of LTC residents with evidence of daytime sleepiness and nighttime sleep disturbance have OSA,[42] with a much higher rate among residents with dementia.[41] Unfortunately, clinicians rarely screen for or document OSA in LTC residents.[43] Unattended home sleep apnea testing using portable monitors is increasingly available for diagnosing OSA, and has demonstrated good sensitivity and specificity for detecting OSA for patients with a high pretest probability.[44,45] Portable, unattended monitoring may be useful for diagnosing OSA in LTC residents who do not have nighttime confusion or dementia. Those with confusion and dementia are likely to remove the portable monitors resulting in a high percentage of missing data. Also, there is a scarcity of data validating home sleep testing in older adults, or in patients with significant medical comorbidities such as chronic obstructive pulmonary disease and congestive heart failure.[45]

In addition to insomnia and OSA, other sleep disorders common in older LTC residents, particularly in those with dementia,[46,47] are central disorders of hypersomnolence characterized by excessive sleepiness, specifically hypersomnia owing to a medical disorder, hypersomnia associated with a psychiatric disorder, and hypersomnia owing to a medication or substance; circadian rhythm sleep–wake disorders such as advanced sleep–wake phase disorder; and sleep-related movement disorders such as restless legs syndrome (RLS) and periodic limb movement disorder. RLS is associated with discomfort in the legs while at rest, along with an overwhelming desire to move while awake. Periodic limb movement disorder is a condition in which involuntary movements of the limbs occur during sleep. Because older LTC residents with dementia may be unable to respond to the RLS diagnostic interview, objective diagnostics are required for this population.[46] Richards and colleagues[26] recently validated an objective RLS diagnostic measure for use in persons with dementia, the Behavioral Indicators Test – Restless Legs. The Behavioral Indicators Test – Restless Legs consists of a 20-minute observation for 8 behavioral indicators and an assessment for the 6 clinical indicators. The frequency of the behavioral indicators (using the hand to hold or rub the leg or foot, rubbing legs or feet together, kicking, flexing against a surface, flexing as if pushing on a gas pedal [like a period leg movement], stretching or straightening legs or feet, crossing and uncrossing legs or feet, and fidgeting) are noted every 2 minutes during a 20-minute continuous observation in the late afternoon or evening. Composite scores range from 0 to 10 with higher scores indicating greater frequency of behaviors. The 6 clinical indicators of history of iron deficiency, discomfort in legs, daytime fatigue, difficulty falling asleep, family history of RLS, and diabetes (negative) are collected from chart review and interviews with patients (if able), caregivers, and family members. A composite score of 2 or more on the behavioral indicators section and score of 6 on the clinical indicators provides good evidence of a positive RLS diagnosis.

MANAGEMENT OF SLEEP DISTURBANCE IN LONG-TERM CARE
Summary and Management Goals

LTC residents (when able), in collaboration their families, physicians, and LTC staff, should together establish goals and strategies for management of each resident's sleep disturbances. Nonpharmacologic interventions should always be considered as the first line therapy. As in community-dwelling older adults, sedative-hypnotic medications should be avoided to the extent possible. In general, both pharmacologic and nonpharmacologic strategies should be etiology and diagnosis directed. Medical and psychiatric comorbidities, and poor environmental sleep conditions and care practices within the LTC settings should be considered as etiologies for sleep disturbances and should be addressed before instituting pharmacologic or other treatments. Importantly, any painful conditions that could interfere with sleep should be evaluated and treated. Evidence-based guidelines, such as those for the assessment and management of sleep disorders in older adults, should guide management strategies.[29,48,49] **Box 2** summarizes strategies for management of sleep disturbance in LTC.

Nonpharmacologic Strategies

Bright light
A number of investigators have examined the effect of increased bright light on sleep and circadian rhythms in LTC settings. Delivery of bright white light was most often by seating participants in front of a light box or by substituting bright white lights for standard wall or ceiling lights in selected areas. The intensity and duration of the interventions varied. Findings have been mixed, and a 2009 Cochrane Collaboration metaanalysis of 10 studies that met strict inclusion criteria concluded that there was insufficient evidence to assess the value of light therapy for people with dementia because too few of the studies were of high methodologic quality.[50] Another review in 2011 by Salami and associates[51] concluded that bright light therapy applied at an intensity of greater than 2500 lux for one-half hour or longer in the morning or all day showed a trend toward improved quality and duration of nocturnal sleep and reduced daytime sleepiness in persons with Alzheimer's dementia. Nine of the 12 studies in the review by Salami and colleagues were conducted in the LTC facilities.[51]

Exercise and social activity
Although light is the most powerful synchronizer of the circadian rhythm of sleep and wake, daytime physical and social activities are also time cues for sleep and wake, and may improve sleep through other mechanisms such as elevating mood. Richards and coworkers[52] conducted a randomized controlled trial on the effect of 1 to 2 hours of daytime individualized social

activity timed to reduce excessive daytime napping for 21 consecutive days in 147 nursing home residents with dementia. Findings included significantly fewer minutes of daytime napping and a significantly improved circadian day–night sleep ratio compared with a control group, but nighttime sleep did not improve significantly.[52]

Two other studies, both using polysomnography to measure sleep outcomes, showed that rather intensive combined exercise and social activity interventions over several weeks improved sleep and other functional and cognitive outcomes in LTC residents. In a randomized, controlled trial in 165 nursing home and assisted living facility residents, Richards and colleagues[53] found that those in an exercise plus social activity intervention group had significantly more total sleep time and non–rapid eye movement sleep compared with control groups. The exercise plus social activity intervention consisted of about 45 minutes of high-intensity strength training (3 days a week) and walking (2 days a week) and 1 hour of social activity 5 days a week for 7 weeks. The exercise plus social activity intervention resulted in both statistically and clinically significant increases in sleep compared with the control group. The exercise plus social activity group also had significant improvements in everyday function compared with the control groups.[54] In another study, 19 residents of a continued care retirement center had increased slow-wave sleep and improvement in memory-oriented tasks compared with a control group after structured social and physical activity for a total of 3 hours a day for 2 weeks.[55]

Multicomponent interventions

A few investigators have measured actigraphy sleep outcomes in clinical trials of multicomponent interventions, most often incorporating reduced time in bed during the day, increased sunlight or light exposure, increased physical activity, consistent bedtime routines, and efforts to decrease nighttime noise, light, and interruptions. The effects on increasing nighttime sleep have been absent or modest; however, there is evidence that circadian rhythm metrics may improve. Alessi and colleagues[56] found a significant but modest decrease in duration of nighttime awakenings and reduced daytime napping compared with controls, but no other improvements in nighttime sleep after a 5-day intervention in 118 nursing home residents. In a subsequent analysis of the data gathered by Alessi and colleagues, Martin and colleagues[57] found an improved rest–activity rhythm with a greater active phase in the multicomponent intervention group compared with the control group. In another study in 173 nursing home residents, Ouslander and colleagues[58] found no differences in sleep measured by actigraphy (or polysomnography in a subsample) between a control condition and a multicomponent intervention that lasted for 17 consecutive day.

Continuous positive airway pressure and other treatments for obstructive sleep apnea

Continuous positive airway pressure (CPAP) is the recommended first-line therapy for the treatment of OSA. Pressurized air through a nasal mask is titrated to reduce the number of events per hour (ie, the apnea–hypopnea index [AHI]) to less than 5, which also decreases sleep fragmentation and oxygen desaturations. A randomized, double-blind, placebo-controlled trial of CPAP versus sham CPAP in community-living persons (n = 42) with Alzheimer's disease and moderate to severe OSA (AHI of 29.8 ± 16.1) showed CPAP adherence levels similar individuals without dementia, and significant pre–post test improvements in the Hopkins Verbal Learning Test and the Trail Making Part B test in those who received CPAP for 6 weeks.[59] In a secondary analysis of the data gathered by Richards and colleagues, combined high-intensity strength training and walking exercise significantly reduced the AHI compared with the control group (adjusted mean baseline 20.2 ± 1.39 vs postintervention 16.7 ± 0.96). The mechanism for the improved AHI may be strengthening of inspiratory muscles.[60] Future studies should focus on the cognitive and functional benefits from treating OSA in the LTC population.

Pharmacologic Strategies

Benzodiazepines (BZDs) are the most frequently used symptomatic treatment for sleep concerns in the older population, including in the LTC setting. However, owing to the unproven long-term effectiveness of BZDs on sleep quality in LTC residents,[61] and the concerns of their adverse effects including acceleration of cognitive impairment[62] and increased risk of falls, the long-term use of BZDs is discouraged in this population. A recent study reported similar shifting patterns of sedative prescription in older adults over time in community and LTC settings.[63] Although BZDs prescription continues to decrease, there is a parallel increase in low-dose, off-label use of other medications with sedative properties such as trazodone and quetiapine, and a high rate of psychotropic polypharmacy.[63] More evidence is needed to support this practice. A systematic review of pharmacologic treatments of sleep disturbances in persons with Alzheimer's disease highlighted a lack of evidence and a need for more trials.[64] Trazodone (50 mg) has some evidence for improving sleep, but the balance between the risks and benefits remains uncertain. Pharmacologic strategies for managing insomnia may be associated with significant side effects and adverse consequences, and should be avoided, or used only when absolutely necessary on a short-term basis. Any pharmacologic treatment should be regularly reviewed.[65]

Complementary and Alternative Treatments

The benefits of complementary and alternative medicine treatments, including dietary supplements, massage, and acupressure, on sleep in LTC residents remain unproven. Additional research is needed in the LTC setting with rigorous study design, large sample size, and both objective and subjective measures for sleep.

Dietary and herbal supplements

Dietary or herbal supplements carry no approval from the US Food and Drug Administration, nor does their production undergo the scrutiny of monitoring by the US Food and Drug Administration. Valerian and melatonin are the most commonly studied supplements for sleep disorders, but quality studies are limited and often offer conflicting results.[66] The potential drug interactions when using supplements remains unclear and may pose risks to LTC residents.[66,67] The prolonged use of valerian has not been well-studied and there is no documentation of extended use in the elderly population.[66] In a multicenter study from 157 individuals with Alzheimer's disease, the use of melatonin did not improve objective sleep measures, although caregivers reported subjective improvements of sleep quality.[68] Safety concerns exist when using melatonin, especially in the elderly, including the potential for residual daytime sedation and prolonged duration of action. When choosing a melatonin supplement for use in older adults, it is recommended that immediate-release formulations be used, with a maximum of 1 to 2 mg administered 1 hour before bedtime.[69]

Massage and acupressure

Research on alternative therapies such as massage and acupressure is sparse. Acupressure has been shown to improve insomnia in LTC residents.[70] A recent review concluded that massage offers a practical activity that could be used to enhance sleep and well-being for older adults in residential care.[71] Positive effects of massage on sleep in LTC residents were demonstrated through improvement in sleep diaries,[72] polysomnography,[72] nursing observations,[73] and fewer requests for sedative-hypnotic medication.[74] However, massage did not reduce daytime sleepiness measured by the Epworth sleepiness scale in a group of adults with complex care needs living in residential care.[75]

IMPLICATIONS FOR RESEARCH AND PRACTICE
Implications for Future Research

More evidence is needed to support the safety and effectiveness of sleep promotion strategies in the LTC care setting. Priorities for future research included testing the efficacy and effectiveness of environmental changes, physical and social activities, and complementary and alternative medicine methods in LTC residents, in studies with high methodologic quality, large sample sizes, and both objective and subjective measurements of sleep and other clinical outcomes. Comprehensive interventions addressing multiple factors that interfere with sleep are likely to be more successful than singular approaches, given that there are multiple causes of poor sleep in LTC residents. Future research should also investigate tailored personalized sleep promotion strategies based on causes of sleep disturbances in individual LTC residents.

Recommendations for Practice

As an attempt to prevent LTC placement, clinicians should assess sleep on a regular basis and closely monitor older adults with disturbed sleep. Education programs for clinicians are needed to develop an awareness of the importance of sleep, and become skilled in sleep assessment and sleep promotion within LTC care settings. As the essential first step to addressing sleep disturbances, sleep should be routinely assessed among LTC residents and considered an important part of care planning. The characteristics and causes of the sleep disturbance must be investigated carefully. Referral for polysomnography or other diagnostic measure is indicated if a primary sleep disorder is suspected. Sleep promotion is a collaborative effort involving LTC residents and their families and care providers. The sleep promotion strategies should be etiology and diagnosis directed, and should not solely depend on pharmacologic treatments.

REFERENCES

1. Who Needs Care? Available at: https://longtermcare. acl.gov/the-basics/who-needs-care.html. Accessed November 11, 2016.
2. Spira AP, Covinsky K, Rebok GW, et al. Objectively measured sleep quality and nursing home placement in older women. J Am Geriatr Soc 2012;60: 1237–43.
3. Valenza MC, Cabrera-Martos I, Martin-Martin L, et al. Nursing homes: impact of sleep disturbances on functionality. Arch Gerontol Geriatr 2013;56:432–6.
4. Alessi CA, Vitiello MV. Sleep disturbance among older adults in long-term care: a significant problem in an important clinical setting. Am J Geriatr Psychiatry 2012;20:457–9.
5. Gaugler JE, Duval S, Anderson KA, et al. Predicting nursing home admission in the U.S.: a meta-analysis. BMC Geriatr 2007;7:13.
6. Blackwell T, Yaffe K, Laffan A, et al. Associations of objectively and subjectively measured sleep quality with subsequent cognitive decline in older community-dwelling men: the MrOS sleep study. Sleep 2014;37:655–63.
7. Diem SJ, Blackwell TL, Stone KL, et al. Measures of sleep-wake patterns and risk of mild cognitive impairment or dementia in older women. Am J Geriatr Psychiatry 2016;24:248–58.
8. Gaugler JE, Yu F, Krichbaum K, et al. Predictors of nursing home admission for persons with dementia. Med Care 2009;47:191–8.
9. McCurry SM, Pike KC, Vitiello MV, et al. Factors associated with concordance and variability of sleep quality in persons with Alzheimer's disease and their caregivers. Sleep 2008;31:741–8.
10. Brinkley TE, Leng X, Miller ME, et al. Chronic inflammation is associated with low physical function in older adults across multiple comorbidities. J Gerontol A Biol Sci Med Sci 2009;64:455–61.
11. Irwin MR, Wang M, Campomayor CO, et al. Sleep deprivation and activation of morning levels of cellular and genomic markers of inflammation. Arch Intern Med 2006;166:1756–62.
12. Neikrug AB, Ancoli-Israel S. Sleep disturbances in nursing homes. J Nutr Health Aging 2010;14:207–11.
13. Kume Y, Kodama A, Sato K, et al. Sleep/awake status throughout the night and circadian motor activity patterns in older nursing-home residents with or without dementia, and older community-dwelling people without dementia. Int Psychogeriatr 2016; 28(12):2001–8.
14. Gindin J, Shochat T, Chetrit A, et al. Insomnia in long-term care facilities: a comparison of seven European countries and Israel: the Services and Health for Elderly in Long TERm care study. J Am Geriatr Soc 2014;62:2033–9.
15. Fung CH, Martin JL, Chung C, et al. Sleep disturbance among older adults in assisted living facilities. Am J Geriatr Psychiatry 2012;20:485–93.
16. Martin JL, Jouldjian S, Mitchell MN, et al. A longitudinal study of poor sleep after inpatient post-acute rehabilitation: the role of depression and pre-illness sleep quality. Am J Geriatr Psychiatry 2012;20:477–84.
17. Goldman SE, Stone KL, Ancoli-Israel S, et al. Poor sleep is associated with poorer physical performance and greater functional limitations in older women. Sleep 2007;30:1317–24.
18. Hahn EA, Wang HX, Andel R, et al. A change in sleep pattern may predict Alzheimer disease. Am J Geriatr Psychiatry 2014;22:1262–71.
19. Alessi CA, Martin JL, Webber AP, et al. More daytime sleeping predicts less functional recovery among older people undergoing inpatient post-acute rehabilitation. Sleep 2008;31:1291–300.
20. Garms-Homolova V, Flick U, Rohnsch G. Sleep disorders and activities in long term care facilities–a vicious cycle? J Health Psychol 2010;15:744–54.

21. Avidan AY, Fries BE, James ML, et al. Insomnia and hypnotic use, recorded in the minimum data set, as predictors of falls and hip fractures in Michigan nursing homes. J Am Geriatr Soc 2005;53:955–62.

22. Nobrega PV, Maciel AC, de Almeida Holanda CM, et al. Sleep and frailty syndrome in elderly residents of long-stay institutions: a cross-sectional study. Geriatr Gerontol Int 2014;14:605–12.

23. Brown DT, Westbury JL, Schuz B. Sleep and agitation in nursing home residents with and without dementia. Int Psychogeriatr 2015;27:1945–55.

24. Dale MC, Burns A, Panter L, et al. Factors affecting survival of elderly nursing home residents. Int J Geriatr Psychiatry 2001;16:70–6.

25. Gentili A, Weiner DK, Kuchibhatla M, et al. Test-retest reliability of the Pittsburgh sleep quality index in nursing home residents. J Am Geriatr Soc 1995; 43:1317–8.

26. Richards KC, Bost JE, Rogers VE, et al. Diagnostic accuracy of behavioral, activity, ferritin, and clinical indicators of restless legs syndrome. Sleep 2015; 38:371–80.

27. Chung F, Yegneswaran B, Liao P, et al. STOP questionnaire: a tool to screen patients for obstructive sleep apnea. Anesthesiology 2008;108:812–21.

28. American Academy of Sleep Medicine. International classification of sleep disorders. 3rd edition. Darien (IL): American Academy of Sleep Medicine; 2014.

29. Gamaldo AA, Sloane KL, Gamaldo CE, et al. Guide to recognizing and treating sleep disturbances in the nursing home. J Clin Outcomes Manag 2015; 22:471–9.

30. Sullivan SC, Richards KC. Predictors of circadian sleep-wake rhythm maintenance in elders with dementia. Aging Ment Health 2004;8:143–52.

31. Lorenz RA, Harris M, Richards KC. Sleep in adult long-term care. In: Redeker NS, McEnany GP, editors. Sleep disorders and sleep promotion in nursing practice. New York: Springer Publishing Company; 2011. p. 339–54.

32. Cajochen C, Munch M, Knoblauch V, et al. Age-related changes in the circadian and homeostatic regulation of human sleep. Chronobiol Int 2006;23: 461–74.

33. Shochat T, Martin J, Marler M, et al. Illumination levels in nursing home patients: effects on sleep and activity rhythms. J Sleep Res 2000;9:373–9.

34. Cruise PA, Schnelle JF, Alessi CA, et al. The nighttime environment and incontinence care practices in nursing homes. J Am Geriatr Soc 1998;46:181–6.

35. Brown CA, Wielandt P, Wilson D, et al. Healthcare providers' knowledge of disordered sleep, sleep assessment tools, and nonpharmacological sleep interventions for persons living with dementia: a national survey. Sleep Disord 2014;2014:286274.

36. Martin JL, Webber AP, Alam T, et al. Daytime sleeping, sleep disturbance, and circadian rhythms in the nursing home. Am J Geriatr Psychiatry 2006; 14:121–9.

37. Pat-Horenczyk R, Klauber MR, Shochat T, et al. Hourly profiles of sleep and wakefulness in severely versus mild-moderately demented nursing home patients. Aging (Milano) 1998;10:308–15.

38. Foley D, Ancoli-Israel S, Britz P, et al. Sleep disturbances and chronic disease in older adults: results of the 2003 National Sleep Foundation Sleep in America Survey. J Psychosom Res 2004;56:497–502.

39. Sahyoun NR, Pratt LA, Lentzner H, et al. The changing profile of nursing home residents: 1985-1997. Aging Trends 2001;4:1–8.

40. Ancoli-Israel S, Clopton P, Klauber MR, et al. Use of wrist activity for monitoring sleep/wake in demented nursing-home patients. Sleep 1997;20(1):24–7.

41. Martin JL, Ancoli-Israel S. Sleep disturbances in long-term care. Clin Geriatr Med 2008;24:39–50.

42. Martin JL, Mory AK, Alessi CA. Nighttime oxygen desaturation and symptoms of sleep-disordered breathing in long-stay nursing home residents. J Gerontol A Biol Sci Med Sci 2005;60:104–8.

43. Resnick HE, Phillips B. Documentation of sleep apnea in nursing homes: United States 2004. J Am Med Dir Assoc 2008;9:260–4.

44. Ward KL, McArdle N, James A, et al. A comprehensive evaluation of a two-channel portable monitor to "Rule in" obstructive sleep apnea. J Clin Sleep Med 2015; 11:433–44.

45. Cooksey JA, Balachandran JS. Portable monitoring for the diagnosis of OSA. Chest 2016; 149:1074–81.

46. Richards K, Shue VM, Beck CK, et al. Restless legs syndrome risk factors, behaviors, and diagnoses in persons with early to moderate dementia and sleep disturbance. Behav Sleep Med 2010;8: 48–61.

47. Richards KC, Roberson PK, Simpson K, et al. Periodic leg movements predict total sleep time in persons with cognitive impairment and sleep disturbance. Sleep 2008;31:224–30.

48. Guarnieri B, Musicco M, Caffarra P, et al. Recommendations of the Sleep Study Group of the Italian Dementia Research Association (SINDem) on clinical assessment and management of sleep disorders in individuals with mild cognitive impairment and dementia: a clinical review. Neurol Sci 2014; 35:1329–48.

49. Bloom HG, Ahmed I, Alessi CA, et al. Evidence-based recommendations for the assessment and management of sleep disorders in older persons. J Am Geriatr Soc 2009;57:761–89.

50. Forbes D, Culum I, Lischka AR, et al. Light therapy for managing cognitive, sleep, functional, behavioural, or psychiatric disturbances in dementia. Cochrane Database Syst Rev 2009;(4):CD003946.

51. Salami O, Lyketsos C, Rao V. Treatment of sleep disturbance in Alzheimer's dementia. Int J Geriatr Psychiatry 2011;26:771–82.

52. Richards KC, Beck C, O'Sullivan PS, et al. Effect of individualized social activity on sleep in nursing home residents with dementia. J Am Geriatr Soc 2005;53:1510–7.

53. Richards KC, Lambert C, Beck CK, et al. Strength training, walking, and social activity improve sleep in nursing home and assisted living residents: randomized controlled trial. J Am Geriatr Soc 2011;59: 214–23.

54. Lorenz RA, Gooneratne N, Cole CS, et al. Exercise and social activity improve everyday function in long-term care residents. Am J Geriatr Psychiatry 2012;20:468–76.

55. Naylor E, Penev PD, Orbeta L, et al. Daily social and physical activity increases slow-wave sleep and daytime neuropsychological performance in the elderly. Sleep 2000;23:87–95.

56. Alessi CA, Martin JL, Webber AP, et al. Randomized, controlled trial of a nonpharmacological intervention to improve abnormal sleep/wake patterns in nursing home residents. J Am Geriatr Soc 2005;53:803–10.

57. Martin JL, Marler MR, Harker JO, et al. A multicomponent nonpharmacological intervention improves activity rhythms among nursing home residents with disrupted sleep/wake patterns. J Gerontol A Biol Sci Med Sci 2007;62:67–72.

58. Ouslander JG, Connell BR, Bliwise DL, et al. A nonpharmacological intervention to improve sleep in nursing home patients: results of a controlled clinical trial. J Am Geriatr Soc 2006;54:38–47.

59. Ancoli-Israel S, Palmer BW, Cooke JR, et al. Cognitive effects of treating obstructive sleep apnea in Alzheimer's disease: a randomized controlled study. J Am Geriatr Soc 2008;56:2076–81.

60. Herrick JE, Bliwise DL, Puri S, et al. Strength training and light physical activity reduces the apnea-hypopnea index in institutionalized older adults. J Am Med Dir Assoc 2014;15:844–6.

61. Bourgeois J, Elseviers MM, Van Bortel L, et al. Sleep quality of benzodiazepine users in nursing homes: a comparative study with nonusers. Sleep Med 2013; 14:614–21.

62. Billioti de Gage S, Begaud B, Bazin F, et al. Benzodiazepine use and risk of dementia: prospective population based study. BMJ 2012;345:e6231.

63. Iaboni A, Bronskill SE, Reynolds KB, et al. Changing pattern of sedative use in older adults: a population-based cohort study. Drugs Aging 2016;33:523–33.

64. McCleery J, Cohen DA, Sharpley AL. Pharmacotherapies for sleep disturbances in Alzheimer's disease. Cochrane Database Syst Rev 2014;(3):CD009178.

65. Anguish I, Locca JF, Bula C, et al. Pharmacologic treatment of behavioral and psychological symptoms of dementia in nursing homes: update of the 2008 JAMDA recommendations. J Am Med Dir Assoc 2015;16:527–32.

66. Schroeck JL, Ford J, Conway EL, et al. Review of safety and efficacy of sleep medicines in older adults. Clin Ther 2016;38(11):2340–72.

67. Shimazaki M, Martin JL. Do herbal agents have a place in the treatment of sleep problems in long-term care? J Am Med Dir Assoc 2007;8:248–52.

68. Singer C, Tractenberg RE, Kaye J, et al. A multicenter, placebo-controlled trial of melatonin for sleep disturbance in Alzheimer's disease. Sleep 2003;26:893–901.

69. Vural EM, van Munster BC, de Rooij SE. Optimal dosages for melatonin supplementation therapy in older adults: a systematic review of current literature. Drugs Aging 2014;31:441–51.

70. Sun JL, Sung MS, Huang MY, et al. Effectiveness of acupressure for residents of long-term care facilities with insomnia: a randomized controlled trial. Int J Nurs Stud 2010;47:798–805.

71. McFeeters S, Pront L, Cuthbertson L, et al. Massage, a complementary therapy effectively promoting the health and well-being of older people in residential care settings: a review of the literature. Int J Older People Nurs 2016;11:266–83.

72. Oliveira D, Hachul H, Tufik S, et al. Effect of massage in postmenopausal women with insomnia: a pilot study. Clinics (Sao Paulo) 2011;66:343–6.

73. Suzuki M, Tatsumi A, Otsuka T, et al. Physical and psychological effects of 6-week tactile massage on elderly patients with severe dementia. Am J Alzheimers Dis Other Demen 2010;25:680–6.

74. Nelson R, Coyle C. Using massage to reduce use of sedative-hypnotic drugs with older adults: a brief report from a pilot study. J Appl Gerontol 2010;29: 129–39.

75. Cooke M, Emery H, Brimelow R, et al. The impact of therapeutic massage on adult residents living with complex and high level disabilities: a brief report. Disabil Health J 2016;9:730–4.

Sleep in Hospitalized Older Adults

Nancy H. Stewart, DO[a], Vineet M. Arora, MD, MAPP[b],*

KEYWORDS

- Sleep • Hospitalized adults • Geriatrics • Older adults • Patients • Hospitals

KEY POINTS

- Despite the need for rest and recovery during acute illness, hospitalization is a period of acute sleep deprivation for older adults owing to environmental, medical, and patient factors.
- Sleep loss in the hospital for older adults is associated with worse health outcomes, including cardiometabolic derangements and an increased risk of delirium.
- Both pharmacologic and nonpharmacologic interventions have shown promise in improving sleep loss for hospitalized older adults.

INTRODUCTION

Nearly 70 million Americans suffer from a chronic disorder of sleep that adversely affects their health.[1] The National Academy of Medicine estimates that hundreds of billions of dollars per year are spent caring for patients with sleep disorders. For example, 1 in 5 of all injuries owing to serious car crashes are owing to drowsy driving.[1] Despite this, most people with underlying sleep disorders remain undiagnosed. Awareness of diagnoses and treatment of sleep disorders among health care professionals and the public remain very low.

Sadly, the patients most at risk for poor, nonrestorative sleep are often acutely ill and hospitalized, when they arguably need sleep to recover from their acute illness. Acute sleep loss in the hospital has been associated with poor patient outcomes, including cardiometabolic effects such as high blood pressure and hyperglycemia, as well as delirium.[2] For instance, Krumholz[3] coined the term "post-hospital syndrome" to highlight the increased risk of readmission for the nearly 3 million hospitalized seniors for diseases unrelated to the index admission. Although studies of long-term consequences of acute sleep loss of hospitalization are lacking, in-hospital sleep loss has been implicated as a potential mediator of post-hospital syndrome.

Prior research has demonstrated that sleep loss is associated with worse cardiometabolic outcomes in the hospital,[4] that hospitalization is a period of acute sleep loss that does not recover in the week after discharge,[5] and that 40% of medical patients without a known sleep disorder are actually at high risk for sleep-disordered breathing.[6] Therefore, the hospital setting is a missed opportunity to optimize the sleep environment for better sleep in the hospital and after discharge, but also to improve diagnosis and treatment of previously unrecognized sleep disorders and potentially reduce unnecessary hospital readmissions.[7]

SLEEP LOSS IN OLDER ADULTS

Changes in sleep among healthy older adults are highly relevant when considering disturbed sleep among older adults in the hospital setting. Sleep in older adults is characterized by decreased

Disclosure Statement: The authors have no relevant disclosures related to this article.
[a] Creighton University Medical Center, 7500 Mercy Road, Omaha, NE 68124, USA; [b] Department of Medicine, University of Chicago, 5841 South Maryland Avenue, MC 2007 AMB W216, Chicago, IL 60637, USA
* Corresponding author.
E-mail address: varora@uchicago.edu

deep sleep (N3), increased amounts of lighter sleep, more frequent awakenings, less rapid eye movement sleep, and less total sleep time.[8] In addition, complaints of insomnia are more frequent in older adults. Older patients are also more easily aroused from sleep by environmental stimuli such as noise or light exposure (which is common in the hospital setting). As a result, sleep becomes increasingly fragmented and sleep efficiency decreases. The circadian sleep–wake cycle also frequently advances with age, resulting in a tendency to fall asleep and awaken earlier, and circadian rhythms are more sensitive to disruption in older adults. These changes occur in nearly all older adults, independent of any medical or psychiatric pathology.[9] Anxiety, depression, loss of social support, pain, and acute illness can all further contribute to sleep disturbances in older patients.

Given the increasing recognition that sleep disturbance in older patients can be considered as part of a geriatric syndrome,[10] it is important to optimize sleep in older patients, especially during times of care transitions, such as admission and discharge from the hospital. Unfortunately, obtaining a good night's sleep in the hospital is often difficult.

HEALTH EFFECTS OF SLEEP LOSS FOR HOSPITALIZED OLDER ADULTS

Although there is a paucity of literature regarding the effects of sleep loss in hospitalized patients,

a model of 2 possible pathways by which sleep loss may impair recovery and function in hospitalized older patients can be proposed (**Fig. 1**). First, laboratory and epidemiologic studies provide evidence to suggest that sleep deprivation itself can lead to a variety of intrinsic negative health consequences (eg, development of delirium, metabolic derangements in blood sugar or blood pressure).[11–14] Interestingly, these health consequences that are linked to sleep deprivation (eg, delirium, hypertension, and hyperglycemia) are also known complications of hospitalization in older patients.[15,16] In addition, these conditions often are associated with administration of additional medications or higher dosages of existing medications for older people (eg, antipsychotics for delirium, insulin for hyperglycemia, or antihypertensives for elevated blood pressure). Furthermore, a significant portion of these medications may be continued after discharge and subsequently result in patient harm.[17] Another possible pathway by which sleep loss can impair recovery in hospitalized older patients is due to fatigue and excessive daytime sleepiness, which may hinder patients' participation in recovery activities (eg, physical therapy), or could diminish patients' desire and ability to be an active participant in their care (ie, ask informed questions, understand medication changes, follow-up tests).[18,19] Understanding this pathway is especially important because diminished daytime physical activity is a

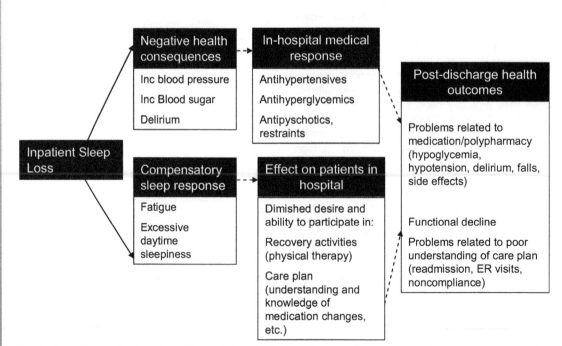

Fig. 1. Potential mechanisms for effects of inpatient sleep loss on older patients. ER, emergency room; Inc, increased.

known contributor to functional decline, a well-known negative consequence of hospitalization in older adults. In addition, hospitalized older patients who are less empowered and informed regarding their hospital care are more likely to experience readmission.[20]

In addition to these factors, sleep loss has been associated with a variety of important outcomes of relevance for hospitalized older adults as they recover from acute illness. In addition to delirium discussed, sleep loss has been implicated in other geriatric syndromes, such as falls, that are also prevalent in hospitalized older patients. For example, in 1 study women with shorter sleep duration or lower sleep efficiency were more likely to suffer from falls in the subsequent year compared with women with normal sleep duration (>7 hours) and sleep efficiency (>70%).[21] In addition, sleep loss has also been associated with impaired immune function in animals and healthy humans, which may have implications for hospitalized older adults.[22] For example, scientists have shown that more sleep after infection yields better survival in fruit flies.[23]

BARRIERS TO PROPER SLEEP FOR HOSPITALIZED OLDER ADULTS

Obtaining a good night's sleep in the hospital is far from easy. Among the factors that are likely to disrupt sleep are environmental factors (eg, noise, light disruptions), medical care–related factors (eg, early morning vital signs, phlebotomy), and patient factors (eg, pain). Patients in a variety of acute care settings report difficulty falling and staying asleep, not feeling rested, increased daytime napping, and a reduction in sleep quality.[24]

Medical Care Interruptions

Frequent awakenings by care providers represent a significant barrier to sleep in the hospital. Patients who are awakened often may be unable to complete an entire sleep cycle, leading to further deprivation of N3 and rapid eye movement sleep. Routine nighttime awakenings by care providers are often used to complete tasks needed for clinicians during the day, such as vital signs or blood draws. Interruptions in observational studies of wards and intensive care units (ICUs) are so prevalent that patients rarely received 2 to 3 hours of uninterrupted sleep.[25,26]

Patient Factors

Issues such as poor health, anxiety, and depression that are often associated with acute and chronic illnesses contribute to sleep disturbances among older inpatients.[27] Studies show that poor self-rated health and the presence of chronic conditions (eg, cardiovascular disease, chronic obstructive pulmonary disease, gastroesophageal reflux, and arthritis) are associated with complaints of poor sleep.[28] Pain is also frequently reported by inpatients as a major cause of poor sleep and nighttime awakenings.[29]

Environmental Disruptions

Hospital noise is more than just an annoyance.[30] The auditory environment should exemplify high and compassionate standards of patient care. Failure to provide patients with quiet rooms affects clinical outcomes through several mechanisms, including increased physiologic arousal and stress responses,[31] medical errors, sleep disruption, and interference with speech privacy.[32] Although the United States Environmental Protection Agency recommends a maximum noise level of 45 dB (dB) throughout the day and 35 dB at night, most hospitals today have noise levels from 50 to 70 dB during the day and an average of 67 dB at night.[33] Medicare has recently made patient-reported noise a publicly reported quality measure as part of its Hospital Compare program.[34] Unfortunately, these data demonstrate that only 58% of hospitalized Americans report their room as quiet at night, which is the worst performing patient experience measure in the entire Hospital Consumer Assessment of Healthcare Providers and Systems Survey. Further, a study in the ICU setting found that 51% of noise was modifiable, with patients reporting staff conversation and television noise as the most irritating disturbances, and interfered with sleep in electroencephalogram recordings.[35] In addition, patients in the loudest rooms get significantly less sleep.[36] In addition, the absence or reduced amplitude of diurnal light–dark cycles in hospital environments can result in disruption of the circadian regulation of sleep.[37] This is especially problematic in ICU settings, where circadian rhythms in patients are particularly abnormal.[38]

PREVALENCE OF SLEEP DISORDERS AMONG HOSPITALIZED OLDER ADULTS

Hospitalization also represents a missed opportunity to screen patients for sleep disorders. The high prevalence of untreated sleep disorders may often complicate or worsen patients' existing conditions. For example, as many as 80% of patients are apparently at risk for obstructive sleep apnea (OSA) according to a recent small single-institution study which screened patients using the STOP-BANG questionnaire.[39] Despite this high prevalence, very few had been evaluated with a sleep study, diagnosed with OSA, or were receiving treatment with continuous positive airway pressure (CPAP) therapy, which is known to improve quality of life and reduce complications.[40,41] The prevalence of insomnia is also high; a recent study suggested that nearly 2 of every 5 patients screened positive for insomnia.[42,43] In another study of hospitalized patients, although one-half of inpatients reported chronic sleep complaints with nearly one-third screening positive for insomnia, there was no mention of a sleep complaint in the admission record.[44] To make matters worse, even if sleep disorders are recognized in hospitalized patients, therapy is often suboptimal. For example, in a nationally representative sample of nearly 300,000 discharges of patients with OSA from nonfederal acute care hospitals in the United States, only 5.8% of patients were identified as receiving CPAP therapy.[45] Given that sleep disorders may exacerbate cardiopulmonary health conditions that actually result in hospitalization, such as congestive heart failure or chronic obstructive pulmonary disease, it is critical to recognize that sleep disorders complicate patient's underlying medical conditions.[46] For example, patients with OSA who undergo surgery are at greater risk of having postoperative hypoxemia, ICU transfers, and longer durations of hospital stay.[47–49] Certain inpatient medical diagnoses, such as acute stroke or heart failure, are associated with a higher prevalence of sleep-disordered breathing.[50–55] Moreover, treatment of OSA with CPAP in patients with post acute stroke or systolic heart failure improves outcomes.[41,56,57] The presence of a highly treatable and very prevalent disorder such as sleep-disordered breathing in such patients warrants a process for better and earlier recognition and treatment.[58]

Perhaps most concerning is that acute sleep loss in the hospital may be associated with the development of chronic insomnia after discharge, especially among those with preexisting poor sleep hygiene.[59] This factor is especially problematic given the association between chronic insomnia and poor long-term health outcomes, highlighting the need for early recognition of insomnia.[60] Last, poor self-reported sleep quality predicts 1-year mortality among older adults who received inpatient rehabilitation.[61] A similar study demonstrated that sleep disturbance as determined by hourly observations of patients in a geriatric hospital were associated with higher mortality at 2 years.[62]

INTERVENTIONS TO IMPROVE SLEEP IN HOSPITALIZED ADULTS

In general, interventions to improve sleep in hospitalized older adults can be classified as pharmacologic or nonpharmacologic interventions. Although some patients do request pharmacologic sleep aids, it is generally recommended that nonpharmacologic interventions be the first line of therapy.[63] In the event a pharmacologic sleep aid is needed, the choice of drug should be customized based on the patient profile to minimize any side effects, especially given the degree of polypharmacy common in hospitalized older adults.

Pharmacologic Interventions

Melatonin
If a pharmacologic sleep aid is deemed necessary, melatonin is well-tolerated and considered by some as the first choice to consider in older adults owing to its minimal side effect profile, low likelihood of drug–drug interactions, and possibility to improve circadian rhythms.[64,65] Small, randomized studies done with ICU patients, hospitalized patients, and in simulated sleep environments showed improvements in sleep duration (as measured by polysomnography) and sleep quality (as measured by actigraphy) when initiating 1 to 5 mg of melatonin at night.[66–68] Although dosing has not yet been standardized, the typical dose is 1 to 3 mg dispensed between 9 PM and 10 PM, depending on the sleeping habits of the patient, and should be given 30 minutes before the desired bedtime.

Sleep aids
Sleep aid medications are commonly prescribed in the hospital setting, although they are generally not recommended owing to concerns about side effects. A retrospective single-center study from 2014 found that, over a 2-month period, 26.2% of patients received a sleep aid, with trazodone being the most commonly prescribed (30.4% of the time).[69] A metaanalysis by Glass and colleagues[70] in 2005 evaluated the risks and benefits of sedative hypnotics in people over the age of 60, and found a statistically significant improvement in sleep quality and sleep duration with sedative use compared with placebo, although the magnitude of the effect was small, and the risks (including falls and cognitive impairment) were great. Although 3 classes of medications for insomnia have been approved by the US Food and Drug Administration (benzodiazepines, nonbenzodiazepines, and melatonin-receptor agonists), 2 of these classes are on the Beers Criteria list from the American Geriatrics Society

to avoid in older adults (benzodiazepines and nonbenzodiazepines).[71,72] Assessing Care of Vulnerable Elders 3 (ACOVE 3) quality measures regarding sleep disorders suggests avoidance of anticholinergic medications owing to their side effect profile. In 2015, the American Geriatrics Society released the updated Beers Criteria for identifying medications to avoid in the older adult population. Medications used for upper respiratory infections such as anticholinergics (including antihistamines) should be avoided.[72] Medications for insomnia such as antihistamines, oral decongestants (eg, pseudoephedrine and ephedrine), and stimulants (eg, amphetamine and methylphenidate) make insomnia worse in the older population, are associated with anticholinergic side effects, and should be avoided.[72,73] Use of other agents as sleep aids, such as tricyclic antidepressants, antipsychotics, atypical antipsychotics, and anticholinergics, should also be avoided owing to their adverse side effect profile.[72]

Pain treatment

The treatment of pain is recommended in the hospital setting, because pain can interfere with the ability to fall asleep, and is a potentially reversible cause of sleep disturbance. Pharmacologic and nonpharmacologic management options should be evaluated for the treatment of pain in the older patient population.[73]

Nonpharmacologic Interventions

Because nonpharmacologic therapies are the mainstay of treatment of sleep disturbances among older adults in the hospital, there is great interest in evidence-based interventions that demonstrate improvement in sleep or related outcomes among hospitalized patients. To this end, 2 relevant systematic reviews have summarized the evidence. First, a Cochrane review on improving sleep in the ICU setting resulted in the review of interventions including ventilator type, eye masks in collaboration with ear plugs, relaxation therapy, sleep-inducing music, massage, foot baths, aromatherapy, acupressure, and visiting time of family members, although the quality of the evidence was low.[74] Another systematic review published found only 13 intervention studies, 4 of which were randomized, controlled trials.[75] Although the evidence was poor, some evidence existed for improving sleep quality, interventions to improve sleep hygiene or reduce interruptions, and daytime bright light exposure. Each of these nonpharmacologic interventions is discussed in further detail.

Relaxation techniques

Several methods of relaxation techniques have been proposed, although the data are limited and quality of evidence is low. A systematic review of nonpharmacologic interventions by Tamrat and colleagues[75] reviewed 4 randomized control trials on relaxation techniques, and found a 0% to 28% improvement of overall sleep quality. A study by Soden and colleagues[76] evaluated the use of aromatherapy, aromatherapy plus massage, or usual care, and no overall differences were found between the groups. When guided imagery for 20 minutes daily was compared with a solitary activity of choice, no difference between groups was found.[77] Last, a study that randomized patients who under coronary artery bypass grafting to 30 minutes of rest, a soothing music video, or 30 minutes of music through headphones demonstrated a 28% improvement in self-reported sleep quality in the group that watched a soothing music video compared with the control group.[78]

Sleep hygiene program

A randomized control trial by Lareau and colleagues[79] evaluated a nighttime intervention of decreasing light and noise, clustering nursing care, and minimizing unnecessary patient contact, compared with usual care. The intervention was associated with an improvement of sleep quality by 7% and a decrease in the use of sleep aid medications. Edinger and colleagues[80] evaluated an inpatient sleep hygiene program to usual care for hospitalized psychiatric patients. The intervention included standardization of sleep and wake times, including removal of daytime napping. The intervention was associated with an increase of 18 minutes (5%) of total sleep time, although neither sleep quality nor significance testing was reported.

Bright light therapy

Three small studies evaluated bright light therapy (3000–5000 lux) use during daytime hours. Mishima and colleagues[81] exposed patients with dementia in a psychiatric hospital to bright light therapy between 9 and 11 AM for 4 weeks, and found an improvement in average total sleep time among intervention patients. Wakamura and colleagues[82] exposed 7 hospitalized patients to 5 hours of bright light therapy during daytime hours, and noted a 7% increase in total sleep time in the intervention arm. Twenty-seven patients with Alzheimers disease were exposed to bright light therapy by Yamadera and colleagues,[83] and were noted to have an increase in total night time sleeping. Although these studies all reported an increase in total sleep time after exposure to bright light therapy, the effects are modest and the strength of the evidence is low based on potential bias, along with measurement and reporting inconsistencies.[75]

Noise reduction

Several studies assessing modalities for noise reduction in the ICU have been performed. These approaches include use of ear plugs in conjunction with eye masks,[84] use of "white noise" (otherwise known as sound masking),[85,86] and the installation of sound-proof materials.[87] The overall quality of evidence with these approaches is also low, and the outcomes used have primarily been subjective sleep measures.[88]

Reducing nighttime interruptions

Two reported studies evaluated the reduction of nighttime nursing interruptions, by altering workflow and reducing patient interactions during typical sleeping hours. These studies suggest that, by reducing nighttime interruptions, there is a reduction in sedatives requested by patients, although sleep duration and quality did not improve.[89,90] Further studies are needed in this area to best determine how to reduce nighttime patient interactions so as to improve sleep quality and duration.

Sleep education and empowerment

In a recent randomized trial, non-ICU patients who received sleep-enhancing tools (eye mask, ear plugs, and a white noise machine) plus education reported less fatigue and sleep impairment than those who just received the sleep-enhancing tools alone.[91]

Multifaceted Protocols

An example of a multifaceted protocol is the "Somerville" approach, where several components were implemented such as an 8-hour quit time, fewer disruptions for routine vitals and medications, and noise control. The investigators noted that fewer patients reported sleep disruption from hospital staff and also fewer patients received as-needed sedatives.[92]

Assessment and Treatment of Underlying Sleep Disorders

Several studies suggest that early recognition and treatment of underlying sleep disorders in hospitalized patients is associated with improved outcomes after discharge. For example, in a very small study, Konikkara and associates[93] showed that, compared with patients not compliant with CPAP therapy, patients with chronic obstructive pulmonary disease who were compliant with CPAP therapy had fewer emergency room and readmission visits 6 months after discharge. In a larger study of hospitalized patients with congestive heart failure, patients compliant with CPAP for a minimum of 4 hours 70% of the time in the first month after discharge had fewer readmissions compared with those not compliant with CPAP therapy after discharge.[94] Likewise, a study of early diagnosis of sleep-disordered breathing in hospitalized cardiac patients using in-hospital portal sleep studies demonstrated that patients who were adherent to CPAP had fewer 30-day readmissions.[95]

SUMMARY

Sleep disturbance is common in hospitalized older adults owing to a variety of factors, including environmental, medical, and patient issues. Sleep loss in the hospital is associated with worse health outcomes, including cardiometabolic derangements and increased risk of delirium. In addition, the hospital setting may represent an important opportunity to identify previously unrecognized sleep disorders, such as OSA, that can impact important patient outcomes. Finally, a growing body of evidence suggests that nonpharmacologic interventions should be the first choice to improve sleep in hospitalized older adults.

REFERENCES

1. Colten HR, Altevogt BM, editors. Sleep disorders and sleep deprivation. An unmet public health problem. Institute of Medicine (US) Committee on Sleep Medicine and Research. Washington, DC: National Academies Press (US); 2006.
2. Pilkington S. Causes and consequences of sleep deprivation in hospitalised patients. Nurs Stand 2013;27(49):35–42.
3. Krumholz HM. Post-hospital syndrome–an acquired, transient condition of generalized risk. N Engl J Med 2013;368(2):100–2.
4. Arora VM, Chang KL, Fazal AZ, et al. Objective sleep duration and quality in hospitalized older adults: associations with blood pressure and mood. J Am Geriatr Soc 2011;59(11):2185–6.
5. Shah MS, Spampinato LM, Beveridge C, et al. Quantifying post hospital syndrome: sleeping longer and physically stronger? [abstract]. J Hosp Med 2016; 11(Suppl 1). Available at: http://www.shmabstracts.com/abstract/quantifying-post-hospital-syndrome-sleeping-longer-and-physically-stronger/. Accessed March 24, 2016.
6. Shear TC, Balachandran JS, Mokhlesi B, et al. Risk of sleep apnea in hospitalized older patients. J Clin Sleep Med 2014;10(10):1061–6.

7. Sharma S. Hospital sleep medicine: the elephant in the room? J Clin Sleep Med 2014;10(10): 1067–8.

8. Wolkove N, Elkholy O, Baltzan M, et al. Sleep and aging: 1. Sleep disorders commonly found in older people. CMAJ 2007;176(9):1299–304.

9. Bliwise DL. Sleep in normal aging and dementia. Sleep 1993;16(1):40–81.

10. Vaz Fragoso CA, Gill TM. Sleep complaints in community-living older persons: a multifactorial geriatric syndrome. J Am Geriatr Soc 2007;55(11): 1853–66.

11. Knutson KL, Spiegel K, Penev P, et al. The metabolic consequences of sleep deprivation. Sleep Med Rev 2007;11(3):163–78.

12. Spiegel K, Leproult R, Van Cauter E. Impact of sleep debt on metabolic and endocrine function. Lancet 1999;354:1435–9.

13. Meisinger C, Heier M, Loewel H. Sleep disturbance as a predictor of type 2 diabetes mellitus in men and women from the general population. Diabetologia 2005;48(2):235–41.

14. Yaggi HK, Araujo AB, McKinlay JB. Sleep duration as a risk factor for the development of type 2 diabetes. Diabetes Care 2006;29(3):657–61.

15. Inzucchi SE. Management of hyperglycemia in the hospital setting. N Engl J Med 2006;355(18):1903–11.

16. Inouye SK. Prevention of delirium in hospitalized older patients: risk factors and targeted intervention strategies. Ann Med 2000;32(4):257–63.

17. Bell CM, Fischer HD, Gill SS, et al. Initiation of benzodiazepines in the elderly after hospitalization. J Gen Intern Med 2007;22(7):1024–9.

18. Ancoli-Israel S, Cooke JR. Prevalence and comorbidity of insomnia and effect on functioning in elderly populations. J Am Geriatr Soc 2005;53(7 Suppl): S264–71.

19. Gooneratne NS, Weaver TE, Cater JR, et al. Functional outcomes of excessive daytime sleepiness in older adults. J Am Geriatr Soc 2003;51(5): 642–9.

20. Coleman EA, Parry C, Chalmers S, et al. The care transitions intervention: results of a randomized controlled trial. Arch Intern Med 2006;166(17): 1822–8.

21. Stone KL, Ancoli-Israel S, Blackwell T, et al. Actigraphy-measured sleep characteristics and risk of falls in older women. Arch Intern Med 2008;168(16): 1768–75.

22. Spiegel K, Sheridan JF, Van Cauter E. Effect of sleep deprivation on response to immunization. JAMA 2002;288(12):1471–2.

23. Kuo TH, Williams JA. Increased sleep promotes survival during a bacterial infection in Drosophila. Sleep 2014;37(6):1077–86, 1086A-1086D.

24. Redeker NS. Sleep in acute care settings: an integrative review. J Nurs Scholarsh 2000;32(1):31–8.

25. Tamburri LM, DiBrienza R, Zozula R, et al. Nocturnal care interactions with patients in critical care units. Am J Crit Care 2004;13(2):102–12.

26. Friese RS, Diaz-Arrastia R, McBride D, et al. Quantity and quality of sleep in the surgical intensive care unit: are our patients sleeping? J Trauma 2007;63(6):1210–4.

27. Beck-Little R, Weinrich SP. Assessment and management of sleep disorders in the elderly. J Gerontol Nurs 1998;24(4):21–9.

28. Blazer DG, Hays JC, Foley DJ. Sleep complaints in older adults: a racial comparison. J Gerontol A Biol Sci Med Sci 1995;50(5):M280–4.

29. Ersser S, Wiles A, Taylor H, et al. The sleep of older people in hospital and nursing homes. J Clin Nurs 1999;8(4):360–8.

30. Grumet GW. Pandemonium in the modern hospital. N Engl J Med 1993;328(6):433–7.

31. Buxton OM, Ellenbogen JM, Wang W, et al. Sleep disruption due to hospital noises: a prospective evaluation. Ann Intern Med 2012;157(3):170–9.

32. Mazer S. Speech privacy: beyond architectural solutions. Available at: http://www.healinghealth.com/images/uploads/files/Mazer_SpeechPrivacy.pdf. Accessed June 1, 2016.

33. Tullmann DF, Dracup K. Creating a healing environment for elders. AACN Clin Issues 2000;11(1): 34–50.

34. U.S. Department of Health & Human Services. Hospital Compare. Available at: http://www.hospitalcompare.hhs.gov/. Accessed June 1, 2016.

35. Kahn DM, Cook TE, Carlisle CC, et al. Identification and modification of environmental noise in an ICU setting. Chest 1998;114(2):535–40.

36. Yoder JC, Staisiunas PG, Meltzer DO, et al. Noise and sleep among adult medical inpatients: far from a quiet night. Arch Intern Med 2012;172(1):68–70.

37. Monk TH, Buysse DJ, Billy BD, et al. The effects on human sleep and circadian rhythms of 17 days of continuous bedrest in the absence of daylight. Sleep 1997;20(10):858–64.

38. Shilo L, Dagan Y, Smorjik Y, et al. Patients in the intensive care unit suffer from severe lack of sleep associated with loss of normal melatonin secretion pattern. Am J Med Sci 1999;317(5):278–81.

39. Kumar S, McElligott D, Goyal A, et al. Risk of obstructive sleep apnea (OSA) in hospitalized patients. Chest 2010;138(4 supp):779. Available at: http://journal.publications.chestnet.org/article.aspx?articleID=1087266. Accessed June 1, 2016.

40. Javaheri S, Caref EB, Chen E, et al. Sleep apnea testing and outcomes in a large cohort of Medicare beneficiaries with newly diagnosed heart failure. Am J Respir Crit Care Med 2011;183(4): 539–46.

41. Kaneko Y, Floras JS, Usui K, et al. Cardiovascular effects of continuous positive airway pressure in

patients with heart failure and obstructive sleep apnea. N Engl J Med 2003;348(13):1233–41.

42. Kokras N, Kouzoupis AV, Paparrigopoulos T, et al. Predicting insomnia in medical wards: the effect of anxiety, depression and admission diagnosis. Gen Hosp Psychiatry 2011;33(1):78–81.

43. Isaia G, Corsinovi L, Bo M, et al. Insomnia among hospitalized elderly patients: prevalence, clinical characteristics and risk factors. Arch Gerontol Geriatr 2011;52(2):133–7.

44. Meissner HH, Riemer A, Santiago SM, et al. Failure of physician documentation of sleep complaints in hospitalized patients. West J Med 1998;169(3): 146–9.

45. Spurr KF, Graven MA, Gilbert RW. Prevalence of unspecified sleep apnea and the use of continuous positive airway pressure in hospitalized patients: 2004 national hospital discharge survey. Sleep Breath 2008;12(3):229–34.

46. Gay PC. Sleep and sleep-disordered breathing in the hospitalized patient. Respir Care 2010;55(9): 1240–54.

47. Kaw R, Pasupuleti V, Walker E, et al. Postoperative complications in patients with obstructive sleep apnea. Chest 2012;141(2):436–41.

48. Liao P, Yegneswaran B, Vairavanathan S, et al. Postoperative complications in patients with obstructive sleep apnea: a retrospective matched cohort study. Can J Anaesth 2009;56(11):819–28.

49. Hwang D, Shakir N, Limann B, et al. Association of sleep-disordered breathing with postoperative complications. Chest 2008;133(5):1128–34.

50. Mohsenin V, Valor R. Sleep apnea in patients with hemispheric stroke. Arch Phys Med Rehabil 1995; 76:71–6.

51. Harbison J, Ford G, James O, et al. Sleep-disordered breathing following acute stroke. QJM 2002; 95:741–7.

52. Bassetti C, Aldrich M. Sleep apnea in acute cerebrovascular diseases: final report on 128 patients. Sleep 1999;22:217–23.

53. Good D, Henkle J, Gelber D, et al. Sleep-disordered breathing and poor functional outcome after stroke. Stroke 1996;27:252–9.

54. Sahlin C, Sandberg O, Gustafson Y, et al. Obstructive sleep apnea is a risk factor for death in patients with stroke: a 10-year follow-up. Arch Intern Med 2008;168:297–301.

55. Oldenburg O, Lamp B, Faber L, et al. Sleep-disordered breathing in patients with symptomatic heart failure: a contemporary study of prevalence in and characteristics of 700 patients. Eur J Heart Fail 2007;9:251–7.

56. Bravata DM, Concato J, Fried T, et al. Continuous Positive airway pressure: evaluation of a novel therapy for patients with acute ischemic stroke. Sleep 2011;34:1271–7.

57. Mansfield DR, Gollogly NC, Kaye DM, et al. Controlled trial of continuous positive airway pressure in obstructive sleep apnea and heart failure. Am J Respir Crit Care Med 2004;169:361–6.

58. White J, Cates C, Wright J. Continuous positive airways pressure for obstructive sleep apnoea. Cochrane Database Syst Rev 2002;(2):CD001106.

59. Griffiths MF, Peerson A. Risk factors for chronic insomnia following hospitalization. J Adv Nurs 2005;49(3):245–53.

60. Morin CM, Benca R. Chronic insomnia. Lancet 2012; 379(9821):1129–41.

61. Martin JL, Fiorentino L, Jouldjian S, et al. Poor self-reported sleep quality predicts mortality within one year of inpatient post-acute rehabilitation among older adults. Sleep 2011;34(12):1715–21.

62. Manabe K, Matsui T, Yamaya M, et al. Sleep patterns and mortality among elderly patients in a geriatric hospital. Gerontology 2000;46(6):318–22.

63. Lenhart SE, Buysse DJ. Treatment of insomnia in hospitalized patients. Ann Pharmacother 2001; 35(11):1449–57.

64. Brzezinski A, Vangel MG, Wurtman RJ, et al. Effects of exogenous melatonin on sleep: a meta-analysis. Sleep Med Rev 2005;9(1):41–50.

65. Zhdanova IV, Wurtman RJ, Regan MM, et al. Melatonin treatment for age-related insomnia. J Clin Endocrinol Metab 2001;86(10):4727–30.

66. Andrade C, Srihari BS, Chandramma L. Melatonin in medically ill patients with insomnia: a double-blind, placebo-controlled study. J Clin Psychiatry 2001; 62(1):41–5.

67. Shilo L, Dagan Y, Smorjik Y, et al. Effect of melatonin on sleep quality of COPD intensive care patients: a pilot study. Chronobiol Int 2000;17(1):71–6.

68. Huang HW, Zheng BL, Jiang L, et al. Effect of oral melatonin and wearing earplugs and eye masks on nocturnal sleep in healthy subjects in a simulated intensive care unit environment: which might be a more promising strategy for ICU sleep deprivation? Crit Care 2015;19(1):1.

69. Gillis CM, Poyant JO, Degrado JR, et al. Inpatient pharmacological sleep aid utilization is common at a tertiary medical center. J Hosp Med 2014;9(10): 652–7.

70. Glass J, Lanctôt KL, Herrmann N, et al. Sedative hypnotics in older people with insomnia: meta-analysis of risks and benefits. BMJ 2005; 331(7526):1169.

71. Young JS, Bourgeois JA, Hilty DM, et al. Sleep in hospitalized medical patients, part 2: behavioral and pharmacological management of sleep disturbances. J Hosp Med 2009;4(1):50–9.

72. Radcliff S, Yue J, Rocco G, et al. American Geriatrics Society 2015 updated beers criteria for potentially inappropriate medication use in older adults. J Am Geriatr Soc 2015;63(11):2227–46.

73. Martin JL, Fung CH. Quality indicators for the care of sleep disorders in vulnerable elders. J Am Geriatr Soc 2007;55(Suppl 2):S424–30.

74. Hu R, Jiang X, Chen J, et al. Non-pharmacological interventions for sleep promotion in the intensive care unit. Cochrane Database Syst Rev 2015;(10): CD008808.

75. Tamrat R, Huynh-Le MP, Goyal M. Non-pharmacologic interventions to improve the sleep of hospitalized patients: a systematic review. J Gen Intern Med 2014;29(5):788–95.

76. Soden K, Vincent K, Craske S, et al. A randomized controlled trial of aromatherapy massage in a hospice setting. Palliat Med 2004;18(2):87–92.

77. Toth M, Wolsko PM, Foreman J, et al. A pilot study for a randomized, controlled trial on the effect of guided imagery in hospitalized medical patients. J Altern Complement Med 2007;13(2):194–7.

78. Zimmerman L, Nieveen J, Barnason S, et al. The effects of music interventions on postoperative pain and sleep in coronary artery bypass graft (CABG) patients. Sch Inq Nurs Pract 1996;10(2):153–70.

79. Lareau R, Benson L, Watcharotone K, et al. Examining the feasibility of implementing specific nursing interventions to promote sleep in hospitalized elderly patients. Geriatr Nurs 2008;29(3):197–206.

80. Edinger JD, Lipper S, Wheeler B. Hospital ward policy and patients' sleep patterns: a multiple baseline study. Rehabil Psychol 1989;34(1):43.

81. Mishima K, Okawa M, Hishikawa Y, et al. Morning bright light therapy for sleep and behavior disorders in elderly patients with dementia. Acta Psychiatr Scand 1994;89(1):1–7.

82. Wakamura T, Tokura H. Influence of bright light during daytime on sleep parameters in hospitalized elderly patients. J Physiol Anthropol Appl Human Sci 2001;20(6):345–51.

83. Yamadera H, Ito T, Suzuki H, et al. Effects of bright light on cognitive and sleep–wake (circadian) rhythm disturbances in Alzheimer-type dementia. Psychiatry Clin Neurosci 2000;54(3):352–3.

84. Richardson A, Allsop M, Coghill E, et al. Earplugs and eye masks: do they improve critical care patients' sleep? Nurs Crit Care 2007;12(6):278–86.

85. Gragert MD. The use of a masking signal to enhance the sleep of men and women 65 years of age and older in the critical care environment. In: INTER-NOISE and NOISE-CON Congress and Conference Proceedings, vol. 1. Institute of Noise Control Engineering; 1990. p. 315–20.

86. Stanchina ML, Abu-Hijleh M, Chaudhry BK, et al. The influence of white noise on sleep in subjects exposed to ICU noise. Sleep Med 2005;6(5): 423–8.

87. Blomkvist V, Eriksen CA, Theorell T, et al. Acoustics and psychosocial environment in intensive coronary care. Occup Environ Med 2005;62(3):e1.

88. Xie H, Kang J, Mills GH. Clinical review: the impact of noise on patients' sleep and the effectiveness of noise reduction strategies in intensive care units. Crit Care 2009;13(2):1.

89. Yoder JC, Yuen TC, Churpek MM, et al. A prospective study of nighttime vital sign monitoring frequency and risk of clinical deterioration. JAMA Intern Med 2013;173(16):1554–5.

90. Le A, Friese RS, Hsu CH, et al. Sleep disruptions and nocturnal nursing interactions in the intensive care unit. J Surg Res 2012;177(2):310–4.

91. Farrehi PM, Clore KR, Scott JR, et al. Efficacy of sleep tool education during hospitalization: a randomized controlled trial. Am J Med 2016. https://doi.org/10.1016/j.amjmed.2016.08.001.

92. Bartick MC, Thai X, Schmidt T, et al. Decrease in as-needed sedative use by limiting nighttime sleep disruptions from hospital staff. J Hosp Med 2010;5(3): E20–4.

93. Konikkara J, Tavella R, Willes L, et al. Early recognition of obstructive sleep apnea in patients hospitalized with COPD exacerbation is associated with reduced readmission. Hosp Pract (1995) 2016; 44(1):41–7.

94. Sharma S, Mather P, Gupta A, et al. Effect of early intervention with positive airway pressure therapy for sleep disordered breathing on six-month readmission rates in hospitalized patients with heart failure. Am J Cardiol 2016;117(6):940–5.

95. Kauta SR, Keenan BT, Goldberg L, et al. Diagnosis and treatment of sleep disordered breathing in hospitalized cardiac patients: a reduction in 30-day hospital readmission rates. J Clin Sleep Med 2014; 10(10):1051–9.

Moving?

Make sure your subscription moves with you!

To notify us of your new address, find your **Clinics Account Number** (located on your mailing label above your name), and contact customer service at:

Email: journalscustomerservice-usa@elsevier.com

800-654-2452 (subscribers in the U.S. & Canada)
314-447-8871 (subscribers outside of the U.S. & Canada)

Fax number: 314-447-8029

Elsevier Health Sciences Division
Subscription Customer Service
3251 Riverport Lane
Maryland Heights, MO 63043

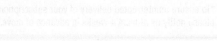

Printed and bound by CPI Group (UK) Ltd, Croydon, CR0 4YY

03/10/2024

01040301-0013